T0292789

Canine and Feline Liver Cytology

Canine and Feline Liver Cytology

Carlo Masserdotti
DVM, Dipl ECVCP, Spec Bioch Clin IAT
Veterinary Clinical Pathologist
Idexx Laboratories, Italy

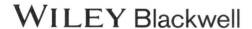

Library of Congress Cataloging-in-Publication Data
Names: Masserdotti, Carlo, 1965– author.
Title: Canine and feline liver cytology / Carlo Masserdotti.
Description: Hoboken, New Jersey : Wiley-Blackwell, [2024]. | Includes bibliographical references and index.
Identifiers: LCCN 2023007030 (print) | LCCN 2023007031 (ebook) | ISBN 9781119895541 (hardback) | ISBN 9781119895565 (Adobe PDF) | ISBN 9781119895558 (epub)
Subjects: MESH: Liver Diseases–diagnosis | Dog Diseases–diagnosis | Cat Diseases–diagnosis | Cytodiagnosis–veterinary | Liver Diseases–veterinary | Liver–cytology
Classification: LCC SF992.L5 (print) | LCC SF992.L5 (ebook) | NLM SF 992.L5 | DDC 636.089/6362–dc23/eng/20230429
LC record available at https://lccn.loc.gov/2023007030
LC ebook record available at https://lccn.loc.gov/2023007031

Cover Design: Wiley
Cover Image: Courtesy of Carlo Masserdotti

Set in 9.5/12.5pt STIXTwoText by Straive, Pondicherry, India
SKY10053839_082323

Contents

About the Author

Carlo Masserdotti graduated in Veterinary Medicine in 1990 from the University of Milan. From 1993, his scientific interest was mainly focused on clinical pathology, particularly diagnostic cytopathology, and he attended specialist courses and institutions in Italy and abroad. He is the author of scientific papers concerning cytopathology and has presented lectures at national and international meetings.

From 1998 he was a teacher and lecturer on the cytology course organized by SCIVAC (Italian Companion Animal Veterinary Association). From 2001 to 2004 he was President of SICIV (Italian Society of Veterinary Cytology). From 2003 to 2006 he was Vice-president of the European Society of Veterinary Clinical Pathology.

In 2005 he received recognition as a Diplomate of the European College of Veterinary Clinical Pathology. In 2008 he achieved postgraduate specialization in clinical biochemistry, at the University of Brescia.

Currently he is a consultant in anatomic and clinical pathology at IDEXX Laboratories. His research is mainly focused on cytological features of spontaneous tumors and inflammatory diseases of companion animals, mainly in hepatic cytology and histopathology.

He enjoys triathlons and the history, art, and architecture of Brescia, his city; he also loves whales as the greatest expression of grace.

Foreword

Veterinary medicine has progressed dramatically over the recent past. Areas of specialization have become more sophisticated and the relevant information complex. Specialization needs knowledge that is focused on a well-defined field to facilitate, through in-depth study, the acquisition of new data. Clearly, this new book by Dr Masserdotti offers a welcome, focused evaluation of the cytological features of the canine and feline liver in health and disease. This work will be a welcome addition to the library and a useful aid for clinical pathologists, clinicians with an interest in cytology, and anatomic pathologists seeking appropriate correlations between cytology and biopsy results.

Diseases of the liver in the cat and the dog span a wide range of possibilities and accurate interpretation of cytological features and correlation with new knowledge of the underlying mechanisms that lead to cytological changes are essential for new understanding to develop. In clinical practice, cytology is a first-line assessment, providing a relatively less expensive or less invasive early look at changes in the liver. Cytology is widely used to establish the presence of liver disease and to determine its nature and often its etiology. Functional tests of the liver can be less informative than desired. In addition, many hepatic functions are secondarily altered, because either hepatic blood flow is impaired or the liver reacts nonspecifically to primary changes in other organ systems. Thus, liver cytology is an essential element in the diagnosis of liver disease. Elimination of the prevailing confusion in nomenclature by consistent use of the WSAVA standard diagnostic terminology, as followed in this book, will assist in reaching reasonable consensus and better communication between clinicians, clinical pathologists, and anatomic pathologists.

This book clearly illustrates the circumstances in which hepatic cytology is sufficient to obtain a diagnosis and those where cytology is the gateway to additional evaluation, whether that involves imaging, additional clinical testing or histopathological evaluation. The features of a broad variety of hepatic alterations are described in focused detail to aid the investigator in the assessment of known liver diseases and the discovery of new disease processes.

This new text will continue the progress of veterinary medicine to serve the management of the individual patient and to expand and enhance our understanding of diseases of the canine and feline liver.

John M. Cullen, VMD, PhD, DACVP, FIATP
Alumni Distinguished Professor of Pathology-Emeritus
North Carolina College of Veterinary Medicine, NC, USA

Preface

Liver cytology is one of the murkiest, most complex, controversial, and difficult topics to investigate that I have ever faced in my entire career as a clinical pathologist.

It is one of the most snubbed topics by anatomical pathologists who tend to boast about their histopathological knowledge, which is considered the only source of information concerning liver disease.

It is one of the most frustrating topics – especially for the novice – to approach when attempting to provide useful data for diagnosis.

Despite some almost insurmountable limitations, over the last 30 years I have come to believe that, despite being an incomplete and often inconclusive diagnostic method, liver cytology has excellent potential to complement and complete the histological diagnosis, especially considering its speed of execution and low costs. In some cases, the latter may even be rendered unnecessary, which benefits the patient.

I thought it might be useful to share my 30-year experience in the management of those liver diseases where cytological evaluation has proved to be an excellent – sometimes conclusive – diagnostic aid, describing, listing, and discussing the characteristics of all those conditions for which histopathological investigation was necessary.

I may be labeled irreverent but I believe that most of what has been written about veterinary cytopathology is confusing, superficial, and sometimes misleading – possibly even incorrect. Among such misconceptions and inaccuracies are historically accepted arguments, such as the so-called "vacuolar liver disease," one of the definitions that have been most abused, often with minimal (if not zero) tangible diagnostic gain, or the claim to apply classic diagnostic criteria – such as anisocytosis or anisokaryosis – to the recognition of hepatocarcinoma. In contrast, in terms of diagnosis of the latter, there is ample evidence of dependence on other morphological criteria.

Before beginning to write this book, I made a promise to myself: "Avoid, as much as possible, any type of psychological subjugation to the data already published and to general beliefs on the subject." The goal was to put across my point of view in the best way possible, at the risk of being considered extreme, and to try to use simple and clear language for the benefit of those who read this book and for those who, in turn, choose the liver as their field of study and research.

I somewhat held back on this revolutionary attitude when I realized that in order to speak in an organic and orderly manner about the liver, I had to follow this consolidated and shared pattern. Therefore, I described the various aspects of liver disease in the same way as the subdivision provided by the reference text – WSAVA Standards for Clinical and Histological Diagnosis of Canine and Feline Liver Disease – which was drawn up by a group of world experts on liver disease, known as the WSAVA Liver Standardization Group.

Obviously, I have appropriately modulated the subdivision of the arguments on the basis of the purely cytological focus of this book. Because of their purely architectural nature, some chapters that are of broad scope and fundamental importance within histopathology, such as vascular disorders, have been excluded, as they are not subject to cytological investigation.

Aware of a certain tendency towards logorrhea, confusion, and the accumulation of data without the order and linearity necessary to be fully understood, I thought of dividing each chapter into different sections: an introduction, a merely descriptive section of the salient cytological aspects of a certain pathological process; a discussion, where I try to put the ideas in order and compare the cytological data with the knowledge already acquired and published; and useful considerations, which are to be used in the report delivered to the clinician.

I truly hope to have created something useful for those who will read my projections.

Perhaps I have written too much and captured too little of what deserves to be dealt with in the context of pathological alterations of cytological samples of the liver. I have certainly repeated myself, possibly because I care greatly about certain concepts, or because I consider some milestone concepts not exactly solid. Many of the concepts I have expressed may be contradictory or controversial, but the liver is as simple in its repetitive structure as it is complex in its morphological manifestations, as well as in the interpretations based on the alterations of its cells. The liver is a questionable topic, therefore I have decided to paraphrase Walt Whitman and conclude with a laconic:

Do I contradict myself?
Very well then I contradict myself.
I am large, I contain multitudes
(Song of Myself, Walt Whitman).

Carlo Masserdotti

Acknowledgments

I would like to acknowledge the people who have helped me understand, write, and correct everything you will find on these pages. Anything that can improve the knowledge of liver cytology of those who read this book is due to them, while any inaccuracy or error is solely and entirely my responsibility.

My heartfelt thanks go to John Cullen. He has been much more than a great teacher, a point of reference, and an inexhaustible source of knowledge. His support in the revision of this book was invaluable. He has become a true friend, and not just a colleague. I have tried to retain everything he has taught me over the years, and I apologize to him if I have not been able to take my knowledge to the level of his teachings.

I would also like to thank Cinzia Mastrorilli for persuading me to consider different points of view, but also for identifying and correcting several inaccuracies I would have missed. She never failed to provide a touch of irony, comprehensive competence, and unparalleled attention.

Lorenzo Ressel is a truly special friend. The ease with which we understand each other is a blessing. His competence and points of view often pushed me to review, deepen, and improve almost every chapter he delved into.

Alessandra Tosini is not only the colleague we would all love to have, but also the one I – undeservedly – am fortunate to have. She was always there, with her patience and tolerance, showing me how to circumvent and solve small (and big) obstacles. Her support was always precious.

A special thank you to Eleonora Piseddu, Ilaria Cerchiaro and to Marcello Garatti for the never-ending discussions and for all they taught me.

Without the help of Cristina Pana, retrieving cytological cases for pictures and comparisons, this entire work would not have been possible: a special thank you for her invaluable support.

Among the many people I need to thank are also those who helped me write this book in many different ways: a simple chat, an opinion, a critical analysis that were very valuable to me in writing this book.

Finally, I thank all those colleagues who, by seeking my advice or opinion or by submitting a case to me, put me in the privileged condition that arises whenever doubts make their way into my head.

Carlo Masserdotti

Dall'esame dei fatti
e dal lor confronto
ho sempre cercato
di discoprire il vero

By the examination of facts
And by their comparison
I've always tried
To discover the truth

G. Ragazzoni

Sordo alle ciance, i miei difetti ascolto
Quelle tralascia e dimmi questi in volto.
Pronto a purgarmi o a confessargli io sono
Chè ragion mai, nè il ver non abbandono

Deaf to the chatter, I listen to my defects
Leave the chatter and tell me (my defects) to my face
I'm ready to purge or to confess (my defects)
For this, I abandon neither reason nor truth

G. Turbini

This book is dedicated to all the people that are seeking the truth

1

Before the Analysis: Rules for Interpretation of Hepatic Cytology

After several years of daily diagnostic practice, I have come to believe that, on the one hand, there is cytology based on classic criteria, which are listed in dedicated chapters of books on the subject, as well as being updated in specialized press articles and discussed at professional meetings. On the other hand, there is liver cytology, which is based on criteria that can frequently differ from standardized, shared, and consolidated concepts applied to several systems. The criteria I am referring to are represented by variations from classic, widely acknowledged issues and interpretations that cannot ignore the clinical context within which the liver disease is being investigated. I believe that the cytological diagnostic approach must be accompanied by in-depth knowledge of microanatomy, as well as cytological and histopathological aspects of the organs being investigated. This statement is particularly important when dealing with an organ such as the liver, since it justifies the differences from classic cytology. Aside from these mandatory bases, I firmly believe there are initial conditions, preexisting situations to the analysis and diagnostic obstacles that must be known in order to modulate one's diagnostic skills. Based on thousands of cases analyzed and diagnosed – frequently supported by histological assessment and further corroborated by clinical course, compatibility with data provided by laboratory and imaging diagnostics or response to therapy – I have been able to draw a few conclusions about the primary skills pathologist must develop to interpret this very complex organ. I have summarized them in a short collection of rules, which I believe should be memorized and taken into due consideration before producing any cytological diagnostic conclusion.

Canine and Feline Liver Cytology, First Edition. Carlo Masserdotti.
© 2024 John Wiley & Sons, Inc. Published 2024 by John Wiley & Sons, Inc.

1.1 The Rules for Cytological Diagnosis of Hepatic Diseases

1.1.1 Rule 1

The diagnostic value of cytopathology in evaluation of hepatic diseases ranges from 30.3% to 82.1% agreement with histopathological diagnosis [1, 2]. This discrepancy is mostly due to the fact that the samples used for cytological investigation represent a very small percentage of a potentially pathological liver, and thus may not be indicative of some lesional processes (low diagnostic sensitivity). Moreover, according to Wang, the diagnostic agreement between cytology and histology should be high in cases of so-called "vacuolar hepatopathy," although this is, in my view, not a specific diagnosis and just morphological evidence of hepatocellular damage. Even a large number of cytological samples from a pathological liver may not detect any alteration, as in some cases of vascular disturbances; in others instances, the tip of the sampling needle collects cells which may not be affected by the primary pathological process occurring or may be affected by aspecific changes. Especially in the course of widespread pathological processes, it is always preferable to sample from many different parts of the liver, as this will increase the chance of collecting samples and therefore data that are morphologically useful for diagnostic purposes. Similarly, when evaluating nodular lesions, comparison between cells from the lesion site and those from the surrounding nonnodular parenchyma may give good diagnostic results (widely described in relevant chapters).

1.1.2 Rule 2

There are some pathological processes, such as amyloidosis or extrahepatocytic cholestasis, whose cytological identification is always extremely useful in terms of diagnosis (very high specificity), even if not corroborated by other tests. For example, amyloidosis in the cat may not be associated with a significant increase in serum amyloid [3]; similarly, cholestasis, in rare instances, may not necessarily be associated with an increase in the concentration of total bilirubin [4]. Indeed, some unmistakable morphological signs may be the result of focal phenomena in a progressive phase and therefore precede certain alterations of other diagnostic parameters.

1.1.3 Rule 3

Many pathological processes can only be successfully interpreted if a histopathological architectural context is available. Furthermore, cytology provides only nonspecific aspects of these processes; for example, fibrosis or inflammation does not provide any information about the causes, extent or distribution but they may highlight an important morphological aspect, which is a valid and sufficient reason to carry out an in-depth histological analysis.

1.1.4 Rule 4

Liver diseases are often not evaluable by cytology. They are often better assessed by histopathology and, in that case, recognition of a specific disease is the result of a morphological diagnosis based on a biopsy of tissue fragments, carried out according to established, accepted, and shared criteria [5]. Cytology is a diagnostic aid that may render histological examination unnecessary (for example, when recognizing amyloidosis or several neoplastic conditions, such as hepatic large cell lymphoma), but in most cases, the information it provides is nonspecific, as in many cases of mixed inflammation or aspecific reversible change. The role of cytology is often limited to excluding other potential suspected pathologies or to reducing or contextualizing the possible differential diagnoses, which must undergo histopathological evaluation.

1.1.5 Rule 5

Sometimes, it is hard not to feel defeated but I will always be determined to persuade clinical colleagues that a morphological diagnosis of cellular or tissue characteristics is, in many cases, impossible without a comparison with all data resulting from clinical and anamnestic investigations, collateral tests, laboratory and imaging diagnostics. The readers of this book will understand that a specific morphological characteristic may correspond to several different clinical conditions (each with its own therapy and prognosis); furthermore, if they have had firsthand experience in making a diagnosis through cytological morphology, they are also likely to understand the importance of being sufficiently informed about data relating to the lesion being analyzed. Given the above, I call on anyone reading this book to join me in this battle: to accept that collaboration between clinicians and pathologists is essential if we are to succeed in improving the management of a disease.

1.1.6 Rule 6

There is an urgent need for cytologists to translate every morphological characteristic of the sample into a diagnosis that is clinically useful in order to come to terms with the relatively scanty information that a liver sample can provide. Cytological samples must be approached with humility, refraining from drawing any diagnostic conclusion when the signs are insufficient or the correlation with clinical indications is incomplete or missing.

1.1.7 Rule 7

Romanowsky-type stains are represented by a group of different stains, such as Hemacolor®, Diff-Quik®, May Grünwald Giemsa and others [6]. These are normally used as routine stains in veterinary cytology, but chromatic results can differ from one stain to the other; consequently, what can stain deeply basophilic or red with one stain can appear as black or brown with another; for example, bile can appear variously as deeply basophilic, greenish or black on the base of the selected stain. Sometimes a color may appear darker or lighter due to the time the slide is exposed to the stains, mostly in cases when a stain procedure is not standardized; always remember that the colors frequently are subjective and must be interpreted carefully.

I believe these rules provide a solid base on which to start discovering the diagnostic secrets hidden in liver cytology. I have attempted to explore them in this book.

1.1.8 Rule 8

Always consider that, after the therapy is initiated according to cytological features, the pathological process can change and histopathologic examination, when done weeks or months after the cytological examination, can result in different findings. For example, an inflammatory process could initially be evident on cytologic preparations but disappear or appear attenuated on histopathologic examination if this latter is done after adequate therapy has started.

1.2 Diagnostic Approach to Liver Disease

In my view, the diagnosis of liver disease is the result of an algorithm that provides an evaluation of the patient based on:

- historical, clinical, and anamnestic signs
- hematochemical investigation
- ultrasonographic investigation
- cytological investigation
- histopathological investigation.

The above is summarized in the diagnostic pyramid shown in Figure 1.1, which clearly shows that only by going from the bottom up is it possible to refine a diagnostic investigation aimed at identifying the causes. Each step contains the indications necessary to proceed to the next diagnostic phase and, eventually, to reach the diagnostic perception of a specific liver disease. With the exception of the first step, which generally provides nonspecific clinical signs, each step can potentially contribute to acquiring information concerning the liver disease in question.

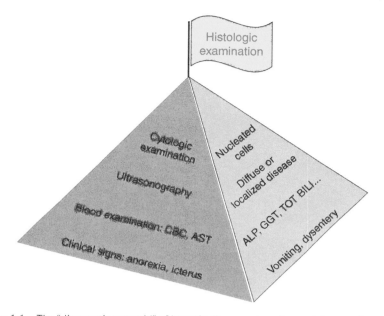

Figure 1.1 The "diagnostic pyramid" of hepatic diseases describes cytology and histopathology as the last steps in clinical, laboratory, and ultrasonographic evaluation and that they need the support of all these data to provide a reliable diagnosis.

In the final levels, cytology and especially histology allow identification of the nature of the pathological process.

1.2.1 Clinical and Anamnestic Signs

The symptomatology of liver disease is generally very nonspecific, as it is represented by generic clinical signs such as malaise, dysorexia or anorexia, vomiting or dysentery. With the exception of jaundice, a consequence of hyperbilirubinemia caused by several liver lesions (may also be caused by prehepatic conditions, such as hemolytic, or posthepatic forms, such as obstructive), hepatic disease has no distinguishing clinical signs. Generally speaking, the symptoms of liver disease are so nonspecific that only an additional assessment (supported by clinical investigation) can confirm with certainty that the ongoing pathological process is localized in the liver.

1.2.2 Hematochemical Investigation

1.2.2.1 Pathological Bases of Liver Damage

When damage to the liver cells occurs, some enzymes contained in the cytoplasm or located on the plasma membrane are released by the damaged cells and consequently enter the circulatory system, a phenomenon that can be measured and utilized as a diagnostic tool if an increase of the said enzymes is found.

The release of cytoplasmic enzymes can result in reversible or irreversible damage. In *reversible damage* (Figure 1.2a), there is a release of small portions of cytoplasm containing the diagnostic enzymes (a phenomenon called "blebbing") even if the cells are not subject to destructive alterations [7]; the small portions of cytoplasm containing the diagnostic enzymes released into the circulatory system undergo lysis and liberation of the enzymes. In contrast, in *irreversible damage* (Figure 1.2b), the release of cytoplasmic enzymes occurs by destruction of the cell (lethal damage), represented by necrosis or apoptosis, although in smaller degree, which results in total leakage of the cytosol into the extracellular space. Detection of increased cytoplasmic enzyme activity (leakage of enzymes) in the serum indicates the presence of damaged hepatocytes (Figure 1.3). Such increase depends on the number of damaged cells, as well as the extent of the damage, so a given increase may correspond to reversible or widespread damage (mild damage involving many cells), as well as to irreversible but localized damage (involving few cells but with severe damage and leakage of all cytoplasmic contents).

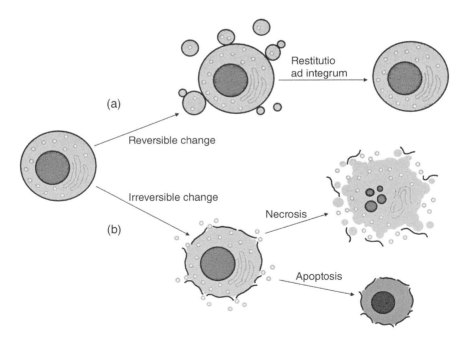

Figure 1.2 (a) Reversible change in the hepatocyte, which recovers completely after the causative process ceases. (b) Irreversible change in the hepatocyte, causing necrosis or apoptosis of the cell.

(a)

(b)

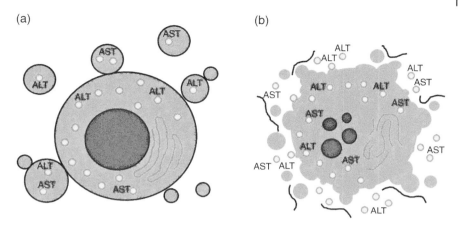

Figure 1.3 Leakage of ALT and AST, which is valuable for biochemical investigation of the plasma, is aspecific and not related to primary causes, since it can occur as a consequence of reversible (a) or irreversible (b) damage of the hepatocyte.

This induced increase in enzymes present in the serum is not correlated to the extent of damage to the parenchyma (focal or widespread). Furthermore, it does not indicate the severity of the damage (reversible versus irreversible) either – it only suggests the presence of nonspecific hepatocyte damage.

In cases of localized irreversible damage, the increase in enzymes may be transitory, although high, since parenchyma is repaired by *restitutio ad integrum*, following substitution of dead cells from regenerative hepatocytes (Figure 1.4a). In cases of widespread irreversible damage, the increase in enzymes may be high and persistent as well, but regeneration is not able to repair the necrotic parenchyma and fibrosis, as a cicatricial process occurs with progression of the damage to cirrhosis (Figure 1.4b). In other cases, an increase in specific enzymes indicates the presence of a pathological process affecting the liver (directly or indirectly), without damage to the hepatocyte membranes. Alkaline phosphatase (ALP) and gamma-glutamyltransferase (GGT) are enzymes located respectively on the membrane surface of the canalicular side of the hepatocyte (mostly ALP) and the cholangiocyte (mostly GGT). Both are released into the bile as a consequence of detergent action of bile salts; both can increase during acute and chronic cholestasis, leaking back into the plasma. There may also be a condition, referred to as "induction," during which the cell produces an overabundance of certain enzymes (inducible enzymes); induction, stimulated by endogenous or exogenous cortisol or many drugs, stimulates increased production of the enzymes' protein via modified transcription, translation or other processes [8]. Such increased synthesis is followed by an increase in enzymes localized on the membrane surface, as well as an increase in the amount that enters the circulatory system.

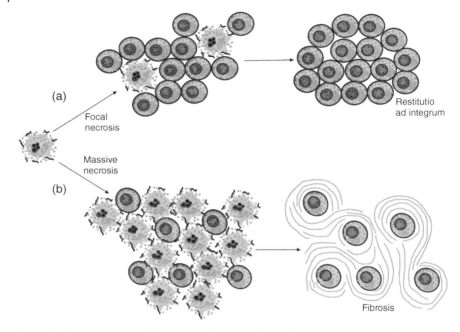

(a)

Focal
necrosis

Restitutio
ad integrum

Massive
necrosis

(b)

Fibrosis

Figure 1.4 (a) When focal irreversible change affects a few cells, *restitutio ad integrum* may be obtained by replacement of dead cells by adjacent proliferative hepatocytes or immature cells. (b) When necrosis occurs extensively, *restitutio ad integrum* is not possible and the only outcome is fibrosis.

1.2.2.2 Diagnosis of Liver Damage

Determination of the increase in the circulation of enzymes used by laboratories to identify liver damage is based on biochemical reactions in which the enzyme being investigated plays a key role. The resulting chemical reaction yields a metabolite whose increase is identified through spectrometric techniques and the concentration of which is directly proportional to the concentration of the enzyme. For this reason, the concentration of liver enzymes is measured in international units (IU), which indicates the activity of the enzyme and not its true quantity, i.e., not in mg/dl. In this respect, it should be remembered that the concentration of a certain enzyme in the circulatory system is a direct consequence of its release, which is caused by either damage to the cell that produces it or the clearance activity of the enzyme itself, which in turn may be altered by pathological processes. It is quite significant how some enzymes, such as lipase or amylase, can increase in the circulatory system not only as a consequence of damage to the exocrine pancreas but also, for example, as a result of alterations in renal excretion function, which is the metabolic process that eliminates these enzymes.

1.2.2.3 Useful Enzymes for Recognition of Damage to Hepatocytes and Cholangiocytes

Useful concepts for interpreting the activity of enzymes include the following.

- Plasma half-life, namely, the survival of the enzyme in plasma. Some enzymes undergo faster degradation in plasma after sampling and consequently, they may appear artificially low and therefore provide unreliable data.
- If evidence of hepatocytic damage suggested by evaluation of biochemical parameters has no correspondence with the cytohistopathological evaluation and vice versa.

Alanine Transaminase (ALT)   A cytoplasmic enzyme resulting from reversible or irreversible hepatocytic damage, whose increase is a consequence of any type of pathogenic insult.

Aspartate Transaminase (AST)   The mitochondrial and cytoplasmic enzyme indicates reversible or irreversible hepatocellular damage but it is also present in the cytoplasm of the striated muscle and therefore, it can increase in the course of muscle damage. To better differentiate the causes of the AST increase, it is advisable to measure creatine phosphokinase (CPK, also known as creatine kinase – CK), an enzyme contained in the cytoplasm of the muscular and cardiac striated muscle cell. Should the increase in AST be consistent with the increase in CPK, the damage is likely to concern the striated myocell and not the hepatocyte. Eventually, *in vitro* hemolysis might cause falsely increased ALT activity.

Alkaline Phosphatase (ALP)   Alkaline phosphatases are a group of isoenzymes located on the outer layer of the cell membrane; they catalyze the hydrolysis of organic phosphate esters present in the extracellular space. At least two isoenzymes are known: intestinal ALP (I-ALP) and nonspecific ALP, with the latter including the ALP isoform of hepatocyte production and that of bone production. Due to its short half-life, I-ALP does not contribute to the serum increase in ALP, which is consequently almost entirely of hepatic (70–90%) and bone (10–30%) origin, with the exception of the so-called C-Canine ALP (corticosteroid-induced ALP), namely the ALP produced by hepatocytes when stimulated by corticosteroids or other drugs (e.g., phenobarbital).

In the liver, ALP, involved in processing bile content, is cytosolic and present on the canalicular membrane of hepatocytes and on the membrane of cholangiocytes. The response of the liver to some primary causes induces an increase in the synthesis of ALP; some of the newly formed enzyme enters the circulation to increase the enzyme activity in plasma. The main reasons for the increase of hepatic ALP are as follows.

- Cholestasis, obstructive (intra- or extrahepatic) and functional (associated with sepsis).
- Drug induction (Figure 1.5), by endogenous or exogenous corticosteroids or other drugs (in dogs).

ALP may also increase as a consequence of bone tissue remodeling phenomena (diseases or bone reworking, growth period of puppies, especially large breeds) or placental production in the final period of cat pregnancy.

Gamma-glutamyltransferase (GGT)   This is a membrane enzyme found mainly on cholangiocytes, as well as in smaller quantities on hepatocytes, exocrine pancreas, and renal tubular epithelium. Its plasma increase is mainly due to cholestasis (Figure 1.6), which is probably secondary to stimulation enhanced by bile acids. Some experimental data suggest hyperplasia of the biliary epithelium as one of

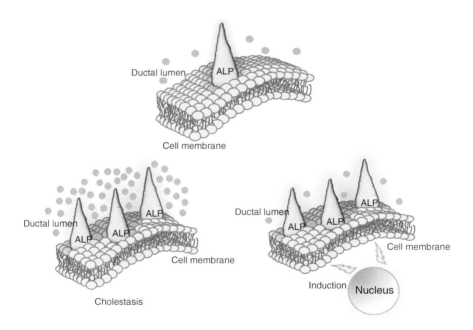

Figure 1.5   ALP is an enzyme located on the external surface of the cell membrane. Many causes, for example cholestasis (left) or induction from exogenous or endogenous steroid (right), may induce increase of ALP molecules on the surface.

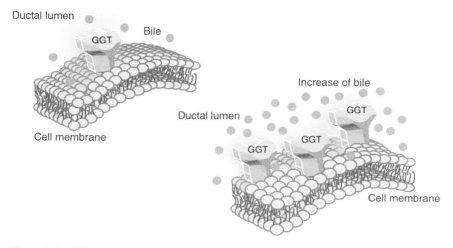

Figure 1.6   GGT, as ALP, is located on the external surface of the cell membrane; many conditions, for example increase of bile into the canalicular surface of the hepatocyte, can induce increase of this enzyme.

the possible causes of this increase. Similarly to ALP, it can increase during pharmacological stimulation or administration of exogenous and endogenous corticosteroids.

Lactate Dehydrogenase (LDH)   Lactate dehydrogenase is an enzyme composed of numerous isoforms and produced by tissues found in several organs, such as the heart, muscles and liver, which limits its use as a marker of liver damage. It may also increase in the course of hemolysis, as it is contained in the cytoplasm of erythrocytes.

1.2.2.4   Liver Failure Diagnosis

Liver damage, whose main evaluation parameters have been listed in the previous paragraph, can manifest as an altered ability of the parenchyma to perform synthesis, excretion, storage, and detoxification functions. Liver damage can alter liver function but if such damage does not exceed at least 70% of its functioning mass, the liver is capable of compensating, showing no alterations and continuing to function normally. If the damage exceeds such compensatory capacity or if hepatic functional mass is decreased, liver failure occurs. In this case, the liver does not fully carry out its normal functions and these deficiencies can be measured with various functional parameters.

Synthesis The liver synthesizes numerous proteins, including albumin, clotting factors, some globulins and lipoproteins; carbohydrates, especially glycogen, the main carbohydrate for intrahepatocyte storage; and lipids, including cholesterol, triglycerides, and fatty acids.

Detoxification Through intrahepatocytic metabolic processes, including conjugation, hydrolysis, oxidation, and reduction, the liver modifies and degrades numerous potentially harmful endogenous and exogenous chemical species, such as ammonium ions, which come from the intestine. Hydrophobic molecules are metabolized to a hydrophilic state for excretion in the bile or urine.

Storage The liver stores glycogen, triglycerides, and trace elements, including copper and iron.

Secretion The liver is involved in some excretory functions, mostly represented by the production of bile and bile acids.

Diseases that can lead to liver failure are not necessarily associated with hepatocyte or biliary damage. In fact, there are serious vascular disorders, such as portosystemic shunt (PSS), in which hepatocellular and biliary damage is minimal or even absent.

1.2.2.5 Parameters of Liver Failure

The substantial difference between liver failure and liver damage is mostly due to the fact that hepatic insufficiency is evaluated on the basis of parameters used to measure its metabolic potential.

- *Reduced synthesis*: decreased concentration of albumin, glucose, cholesterol, and fibrinogen in plasma.
- *Reduced detoxification capacity*: hyperammonemia is one of the most common alterations of this function, which is the result of the liver's inability to metabolize intestinal-derived ammonia.
- *Alterations in secretion*: bile is an important metabolite that is secreted by the liver. Restriction of secretion or retention of bile can occur, due to the conditions described below in relation to jaundice, as well as obstructive events affecting the biliary outflow.

Bilirubin Bilirubin is a catabolism derivative of the heme molecule and, to a small extent, of myoglobin or other enzymes, such as cytochromes. The liver captures the circulating bilirubin bound to albumin (called nonconjugated) and combines it with glucuronic acid (conjugated bilirubin), a process by which, after becoming water soluble, it is eliminated with the bile salts into the bile. Increase in plasma bilirubin may be the result of increased production (hemolysis), decreased hepatocyte capacity to capture or eliminate bilirubin, or occlusion of biliary outflow.

Urea The liver metabolizes ammonium ion and transforms it into urea; hypoazotemia may occur as a consequence of hepatic failure, hepatocellular diseases, portosystemic shunts or urea cycle enzyme deficiencies.

Ammonium Hyperammonemia may occur as a result of decreased clearance from portal blood or due to a decrease of functional hepatic mass, mostly as in diffuse hepatocellular disease, congenital or acquired portosystemic shunt.

Albumin Albumin is synthesized by the hepatocyte and has a long plasma half-life (8.2 days in dogs [9]); its decrease can be associated with chronic hepatic insufficiency.

Cholesterol The liver synthesizes cholesterol and the proteins necessary for its plasma transport. Hypocholesterolemia can be associated with forms of severe insufficiency.

Proteins Involved in Coagulation Pro- and anticoagulant proteins are synthesized by the liver, therefore hepatic failure can lead to disturbed clotting.

Glucose Glucose is stored by the liver in the form of glycogen and released when needed. Consequently, hepatic insufficiency can be associated with forms of moderate hypoglycemia, a consequence of decreased gluconeogenesis activity.

Bile Acids Bile acids are synthesized by the liver and released with the bile. They are reabsorbed in the intestine by the portal circulation and subsequently transported back to the liver, with the exception of a small amount which remains in the circulating blood and is eliminated with the urine or stool.
Abnormal biliary acid levels can be assessed in two ways.

- *Measurement of pre- and postprandial bile acids*: this is an effective way to compare the amount of bile acids in the circulation in a fasting state compared to levels following gallbladder emptying. Abnormally high postprandial levels indicate that the liver cannot clear the bile acids, due to either shunting of portal blood or hepatocyte injury. High fasting bile acid levels are also an indication of shunting of portal blood or hepatic failure. Obtaining unambiguous data may be difficult.

- *Levels of urinary bile acids*: the one-time collection of urine, compared to fasting and postprandial blood collection, makes this assay attractive for assessing bile acids.

1.2.3 Ultrasonographic Investigation

When the presence of a liver disease can be ascertained through the diagnostic investigations listed above, evaluation of the parenchyma through diagnostic imaging becomes essential, as this can establish the type of lesions on the hepatic parenchyma or biliary tree. A complete and exhaustive evaluation of ultrasonographic diagnostics and its merits is beyond the purpose of this book so I will only underline the key role of diagnostic imaging, especially when it is necessary to identify characteristics that, in turn, render subsequent investigations necessary.

Ultrasonographic examinations allow us to establish the existence of a pathological process spreading to the whole parenchyma, as in the course of suspicious pathological accumulations of lipids or glycogen [10]. This investigation is crucial, especially if performed with Doppler and contrast ultrasonography, as it identifies portal circulation disorders, such as PSS [11]. Ultrasonographic examination allows us to highlight the presence of nodular lesions, such as in the course of primary or metastatic neoplasia and even with the contrast-enhanced ultrasonography (CEUS) method, and investigate the vascular characteristics of some nodular lesions, as well as to correlate the pattern to any malignant behavior [12].

In addition, ultrasonographic examination can identify peculiar characteristics of biliary swelling and primary diseases, such as cystic hyperplasia of the gallbladder. Although ultrasonographic investigations rarely result in conclusive diagnoses, the value of this tool is undeniable, especially its ability to establish whether the liver damage is widespread or localized and, consequently, to identify possible differential diagnoses. Ultrasonographic examination is also an essential support for subsequent cytological or histopathological analysis; depending on the appearance of the lesion found, it is possible to sample by means of fine needle capillary suction (FNCS) both the parenchyma affected by widespread processes and nodular lesions, even those of small dimensions, as this technique allows us to target precise parts of the parenchyma.

Finally, the use of ultrasonography for sampling the hepatic parenchyma with a cutting needle allows us, on the one hand, to obtain suitable samples for histopathological investigation and, on the other, to monitor any hemorrhagic incidents.

1.2.4 Cytological and Histopathological Investigation

If a diagnosis has not been made, the progression upward through the levels of the diagnostic pyramid (Figure 1.1) ultimately results in morphological assessments of the lesion process based on cytological observations, which are widely discussed in this book using histological terminology, which has only been touched upon in some chapters and is abundantly dealt with in the material included in the references.

1.2.4.1 Sample Collection

While an extensive review of sampling methods is beyond the scope of this book, a brief summary of sampling issues should be useful for the reader. Given that the target audience of this book is the skilled and expert cytologist, I will not provide a complete description of the sampling process, which is already extensively described in available cytology books.

Fine needle aspiration (FNA) is widely used to collect cytology samples, usually performed using a 6 or 12 cc syringe and a 22 gauge, 1.5 to 3.5 in. disposable hypodermic or spinal needle. FNCS [13], conducted with ultrasonographic guidance (Figure 1.7), is widely used to collect cytology samples from the liver, typically using a 25 gauge, 1.5 to 3.5 in. disposable hypodermic or spinal needle. Although

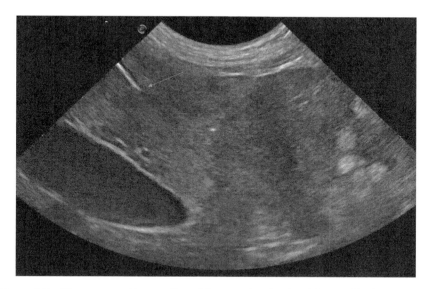

Figure 1.7 Ultrasonographic sampling of liver; notice the tip of the needle that enters the parenchyma (yellow arrow).

FNA has been used for a long time, FNCS is my preferred method of collection because of the high number of cells retrieved, the integrity of arrangements, and the minimal blood contamination.

The needle is inserted into the liver via a percutaneous transabdominal approach in small animals or transthoracically in large animals. FNA, FNCS, Tru-Cut®, and Menghini needles, laparoscopic forceps, and surgical wedge biopsy can all be used to sample hepatic tissue, the former by direct smear of the sample, the others by touch imprint of the sampled hepatic tissue on a slide [14]. Large-scale studies of complications associated with liver aspirates in dogs, cats, and horses are lacking, although hemorrhage and accidental perforation of large biliary ducts or the gallbladder are possible [15]. A small amount of blood loss is always expected, which can be visualized ultrasonographically or during laparoscopy or surgery. The average amount of blood loss from a liver biopsy is reported to be around 2 ml in healthy dogs [15, 16]. The risk for prolonged or excessive bleeding should be assessed by evaluating coagulation times before performing the procedure [17, 18]. Studies of ultrasound-guided and laparoscopic liver biopsies in dogs, cats, and horses suggest that this procedure is generally safe [19, 20].

1.2.4.2 Cytological Approach to Hepatic Diseases

Clinical pathologists should always bear in mind that cytology should be considered a preliminary evaluation of hepatic diseases and that cytological sampling may produce one of the following outcomes.

- *Nondiagnostic*: many cytological samples, on the basis of the previously discussed rules, are not useful for diagnosis, mostly because the primary disease site has not been sampled or because architectural or vascular changes are not evaluable. In these cases, just a description of the aspecific changes of hepatocytes, inflammatory conditions or other aspecific changes should be given in the report.
- *Suggestive of differential diagnosis*: in some cases, although not definitively diagnostic, cytological changes may be indicative of a specific pathological process, as for example the presence of fibrosis or cholestasis, although histopathological investigation is necessary to correctly address this change.
- *Diagnostic*: in some cases, cytology is definitively diagnostic and histopathological investigation is not necessary to correctly manage the patient, for example in cases of amyloidosis or in many cases of primary or metastatic neoplasm.

1.3   Key Points

- Liver diseases can be correctly identified only if all data, from clinical, historical, laboratory, and ultrasonographic investigations, are available.
- Clinical data are mostly aspecific.

- Biochemical abnormalities are mostly represented by increased plasma concentrations of ALT, AST, ALP, GGT, and total bilirubin, that are the most useful biochemical parameters to recognize a hepatic disease.
- Liver can be affected by diffuse or focal pathological processes; these processes may be recognized by ultrasonographic investigation.
- Cells sampled by cytological methods can be diagnostic, helpful for final diagnosis or aspecific; this diagnostic power is correlated with the nature of the primary process.
- Diagnostic power may also be correlated with the likelihood that the tip of the needle samples an area where a primary pathological process occurs and with the number, appearance, and integrity of diagnostic cells.

References

1 Wang, K.Y., Panciera, D.L., Al-Rukibat, R.K., and Radi, Z.A. (2004). Accuracy of ultrasound-guided fine-needle aspiration of the liver and cytologic findings in dogs and cats: 97 cases (1990–2000). *J. Am. Vet. Med. Assoc.* 224 (1): 75–78.

2 Roth, L. (2001). Comparison of liver cytology and biopsy diagnoses in dogs and cats: 56 cases. *Vet. Clin. Pathol.* 30 (1): 35–38.

3 Neo-Suzuki, S., Mineshige, T., Kamiie, J. et al. (2017). Hepatic AA amyloidosis in a cat: cytologic and histologic identification of AA amyloid in macrophages. *Vet. Clin. Pathol.* 46 (2): 331–336.

4 Fahie, M.A. and Martin, R.A. (1995). Extrahepatic biliary tract obstruction: a retrospective study of 45 cases (1983–1993). *J. Am. Anim. Hosp. Assoc.* 31 (6): 478–482.

5 Rothuizen, J., Desmet, V.J., Van den Ingh, T.S.G.A.M. et al. (2006). Sampling and handling of liver tissue. In: *Standard for Clinical and Histological Diagnosis of Canine and Feline Liver Disease* (ed. WSAVA Liver Standardization Group), 5–14. St Louis, MO: Saunders.

6 Krafts, K.P. and Pambuccian, S.E. (2011). Romanowsky staining in cytopathology: history, advantages and limitations. *Biotech. Histochem.* 86 (2): 82–93.

7 Stockham, S.L. and Scott, M.A. (2008). Enzymes. In: *Fundamentals of Clinical Pathology*, 2e (ed. S.L. Stockham and M.A. Scott), 642–643. Ames, IA: Wiley Blackwell.

8 Stockham, S.L. and Scott, M.A. (2008). Enzymes. In: *Fundamentals of Clinical Pathology*, 2e (ed. S.L. Stockham and M.A. Scott), 644–645. Ames, IA: Wiley Blackwell.

9 Stockham, S.L. and Scott, M.A. (2008). Proteins. In: *Fundamentals of Clinical Pathology*, 2e (ed. S.L. Stockham and M.A. Scott), 371. Ames, IA: Wiley Blackwell.

10 Feeney, D.A., Anderson, K.L., Ziegler, L.E. et al. (2008). Statistical relevance of ultrasonographic criteria in the assessment of diffuse liver disease in dogs and cats. *Am. J. Vet. Res.* 69 (2): 212–221.

11 D'Anjou, M.A., Penninck, D., Cornejo, L., and Pibarot, P. (2004). Ultrasonographic diagnosis of portosystemic shunting in dogs and cats. *Vet. Radiol. Ultrasound* 45 (5): 424–437.

12 Kanemoto, H., Ohno, K., Nakashima, K. et al. (2009). Characterization of canine focal liver lesions with contrast-enhanced ultrasound using a novel contrast agent-sonazoid. *Vet. Radiol. Ultrasound* 50 (2): 188–194.

13 Mair, S., Dunbar, F., Becker, P.J., and Du Plessis, W. (1989). Fine needle cytology – is aspiration suction necessary? A study of 100 masses in various sites. *Acta Cytol.* 33 (6): 809–813.

14 Kerwin, S.C. (1995). Hepatic aspiration and biopsy techniques. *Vet. Clin. North Am. Small Anim. Pract.* 25 (2): 275–291.

15 Rawlings, C.A. and Howerth, E.W. (2004). Obtaining quality biopsies of the liver and kidney. *J. Am. Anim. Hosp. Assoc.* 40 (5): 352–352.

16 Vasanjee, S.C., Bubenik, L.J., Hosgood, G. et al. (2006). Evaluation of hemorrhage, sample size, and collateral damage for five hepatic biopsy methods in dogs. *Vet. Surg.* 35 (1): 86–93.

17 Bigge, L.A., Brown, D.J., and Penninck, D.G. (2001). Correlation between coagulation profile findings and bleeding complications after ultrasound-guided biopsies: 434 cases. *J. Am. Anim. Hosp. Assoc.* 37 (3): 228–233.

18 Johns, I.C. and Sweeney, R.W. (2008). Coagulation abnormalities and complications after percutaneous liver biopsy in horses. *J. Vet. Intern. Med.* 22 (1): 185–189.

19 Petre, S.L., McClaran, J.K., Bergman, P.J. et al. (2012). Safety and efficacy of laparoscopic hepatic biopsy in dogs: 80 cases (2004–2009). *J. Am. Vet. Med. Assoc.* 240 (2): 181–185.

20 McDevitt, H.L., Mayhew, P.D., Giuffrida, M.A. et al. (2016). Short-term clinical outcome of laparoscopic liver biopsy in dogs: 106 cases (2003–2013). *J. Am. Vet. Med. Assoc.* 248 (1): 83–90.

2

Normal Histology and Cytology of the Liver

I would like to begin this long journey into the world of hepatic cytology by specifying that a correct interpretation of the pathological characteristics of the cells contained in tissue is impossible without a deep understanding of "normal" cells, in particular their characteristics and microanatomical arrangement within the tissue itself. Comprehensive knowledge of what is "normal" is crucial to identifying what is "not normal," and therefore to recognizing the pathological aspects. This analysis will demonstrate that the difference between a normal and a pathological state is at times very subtle; furthermore, in some cases, only comparison with an actual clinical or symptomatic state can lead to the suggestion of primary or secondary pathological processes.

2.1   Normal Histology of the Liver

In order to allow adaptation to size variations during large organic functions, the liver is subdivided into distinct lobes; each lobe is subdivided into multi-unit structures called **hepatic lobules** [1] (Figures 2.1 and 2.2).

Each polygonally shaped lobule receives vascular ramifications located at its vertices, represented by ramifications of the portal vein, which carry blood from the gastrointestinal tract, spleen, and pancreas (over 80% of the blood entering the liver), and of the hepatic artery that carries oxygenated blood from the aorta (Figures 2.3 and 2.4). The portal vascular arrangement is necessary for liver functions including detoxification, nutrition, and microbiological clearance, and for the supply of oxygen as well. Each lobule includes radiated trabeculae of hepatocytes which converge from the periphery of the polygon toward the center, which is represented by the centrilobular vein (Figure 2.5).

From the ramifications of the portal vein and hepatic artery, which terminate in the portal tracts (consisting of a more or less expanded stromal support),

Canine and Feline Liver Cytology, First Edition. Carlo Masserdotti.
© 2024 John Wiley & Sons, Inc. Published 2024 by John Wiley & Sons, Inc.

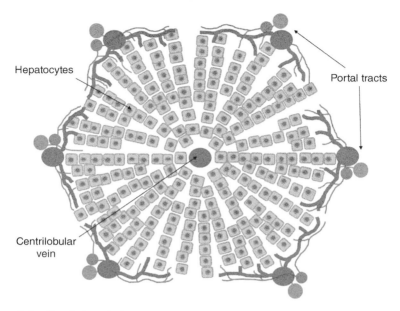

Hepatocytes

Portal tracts

Centrilobular
vein

Figure 2.1   Classic hepatic lobule, with hexagonal shape.

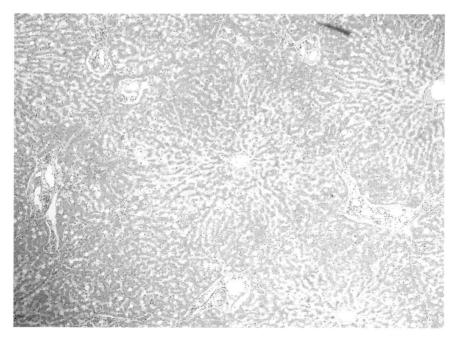

Figure 2.2   Normal liver, dog. Histological section of classic hepatic lobule: notice the six-sided arrangement of hepatocytes centered on the hepatic vein and peripherally demarcated by portal tracts (HE, 10×).

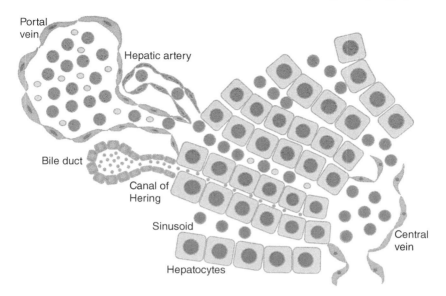

Figure 2.3 The drawing shows a selected section of the classic lobule, with the portal-centrolobular disposition of vessels, hepatocytes, and biliary ducts.

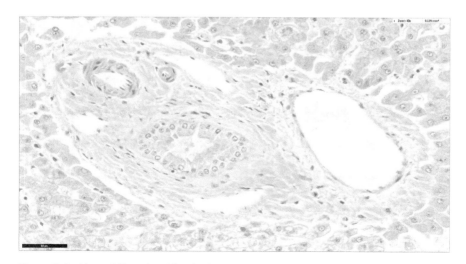

Figure 2.4 Normal liver, dog. Histological section of a normal portal tract (HE, 40×).

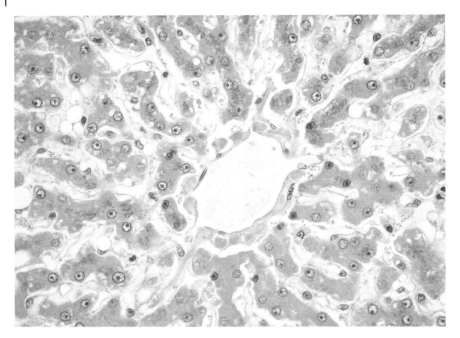

Figure 2.5   Normal liver, dog. Histological section of a centrilobular area; notice the radiate organization of sinusoids, directed from the portal tract toward the central vein (HE, 40×).

the blood, in correspondence with the first hepatocyte row (called the **limiting plate**), mixes before entering the sinusoid capillaries. From here, it begins to flow, bathing the surface of the hepatocyte trabeculae (Figures 2.6 and 2.7) and merging in the centrilobular area, where it is collected and carried out of the liver by the hepatic vein. Sinusoid capillaries are delimited by specific endotheliocytes, whose fenestrated cytoplasm allows the passage of solutes and plasma molecules with a diameter of up to approximately 1000 Å. Free of basement-like membrane, sinusoid capillaries separate the blood flow from the hepatocyte rows by interposition of a thin cavity, the **space of Disse**. This gap is supported by a minimum quantity of collagen fibrils (mostly type IV collagen and laminin), as well as by molecules of proteoglycans or glycoproteins, such as fibronectin and laminin, generally named the extracellular matrix (ECM). Through these very thin barriers, metabolic exchanges take place between the portal blood and the mixed arterial blood and hepatocytes, which receive nutritional substances, metabolites and oxygen; hepatocytes contain a large number of enzymes able to break down and metabolize most of what has been absorbed.

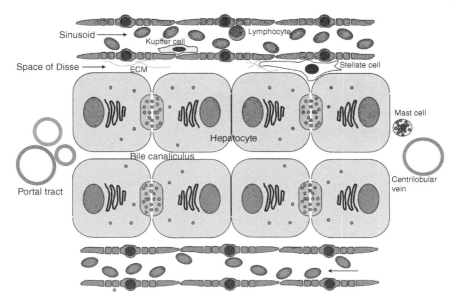

Figure 2.6 Schematic representation of hepatic rows, separated by canalicular space and delimited by the space of Disse and sinusoidal endothelial cells. The image also shows the localization of nonhepatic liver cells.

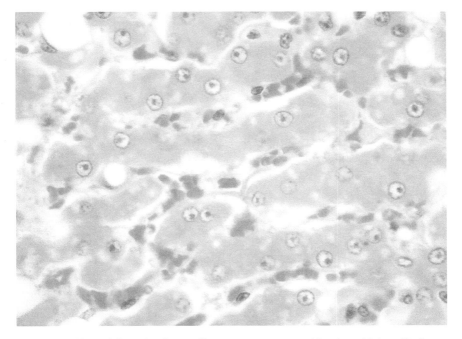

Figure 2.7 Normal liver, dog. Rows of hepatocytes, separated by sinusoidal capillaries (HE, 100×).

In terms of pathophysiology, the fact that through the portal blood, the hepatocytes also receive bacteria coming from the intestine or potentially toxic molecules is also of key importance. After receiving and metabolizing all the substances coming from the portal and arterial blood, the hepatocytes transfer the results of synthesis or detoxification into the circulation through the venous system. The Kupffer cells, found close to the space of Disse and intercalated with the sinusoidal endothelial cells, are the specialized macrophages of the hepatic parenchyma with mostly immune surveillance functions. Under normal conditions, they can also phagocytize bacteria coming especially from blood or toxic macromolecules. Stellate cells (also called Ito cells) in the space of Disse are cytoplasmic elements with elongated extensions, which protrude into the interstitium and sometimes cross the sinusoidal lumen. The main role of these cells is storing vitamin A and producing the ECM on which endotheliocytes rest. Some rare lymphocytes may be found near the endotheliocytes or between the hepatocyte rows, while some mast cells may be located near the centrilobular venous vessel, as demonstrated in dogs.

Hepatocytes are organized in coupled rows delimited by the sinusoid capillaries (as previously described). These rows create a narrow space called the **biliary canaliculus,** which is in direct contact with the membrane of the hepatocyte, which secretes bile, the main metabolic product of the liver. The bile goes into the bloodstream and reaches the thin canaliculi up to the last tract, which is normally referred to as the **Hering canal**. Finally, it enters the **bile ducts**, which are delimited by a single line of cholangiocytes – cuboidal cells resting on a basal membrane. In correspondence with this transition area are the progenitor cells (or **oval cells)** which are not morphologically recognizable, capable of totipotent differentiation and transformation into both hepatocytes and cholangiocytes. From the distal to the intermediate portal spaces, the smaller bile ducts become progressively larger, forming the large bile ducts, delimited by columnar cells and ending in the **choledochus**.

In cats and dogs, there is a saccular diverticulum of the choledochus, the **gallbladder**. This consists of a sack-like organ, located between the quadrate and right medial liver lobes, with a vascularized fibromuscular wall, capable of contraction and delimited luminally by columnar epithelium, organized in papillary projections and tubular structures. Its blood supply is only provided by an artery derived from the left hepatic artery, making the wall susceptible to ischemic necrosis if this vessel becomes compromised. The function of the gallbladder is the storage of bile, that may be acidified by epithelial secretions or modified by addition of mucin. The gallbladder is connected by a short cystic duct to the common bile duct (choledochus) that ends in the **duodenal papilla**, through which the bile flows into the intestinal lumen. In cats, the choledochus joins the pancreatic duct before ending in the duodenal papilla.

On the basis of the hepatocyte distribution – within the imaginary polygon between the vertices of the portal spaces and the center (represented by the centrilobular vein and the rays, which are constituted by the imaginary chains) – some representations of the functional unit of the liver have been formulated. The **classic hepatic lobule**, represented by the described polygon, constitutes a purely microanatomic entity; from a functional and metabolic point of view, it was formulated by Rappaport as a rhomboidal anatomical unit, named the **hepatic acinus** or **Rappaport acinus** [2] (Figures 2.8–2.10), represented by four vertices, two portal spaces and two centrilobular vessels (opposite two by two), whose presence may be useful to identify pathophysiological events involving the liver.

On the basis of this subdivision, it is clear how the blood coming out of the portal section crosses three distinct common areas belonging to two classic lobules. **Zone 1** (or **periportal zone**), located near the portal space, is the first to receive oxygenated blood, but it is also the first to receive any toxic metabolites. Selectively localized damage to this area may be mediated by the action of a toxic molecule or etiological agent. **Zone 3** (or **centrilobular zone**) is the last to receive oxygenated

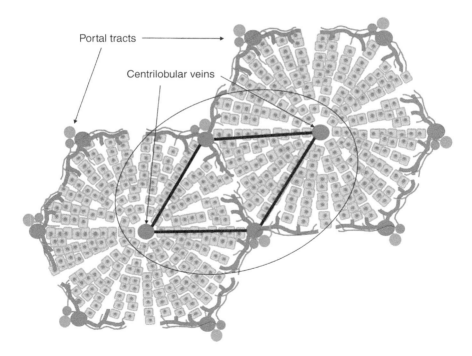

Figure 2.8 Schematic representation of the Rappaport acinus; two adjacent classic lobules form a polygonal area with two portal tract and two centrolobular veins.

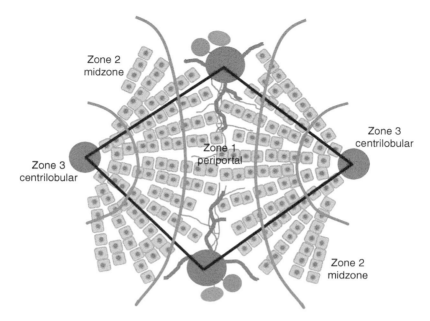

Figure 2.9 Schematic representation of the distribution of functional areas in the Rappaport acinus, subdivided into zone 1 (periportal), zone 2 (midzonal), and zone 3 (centrilobular).

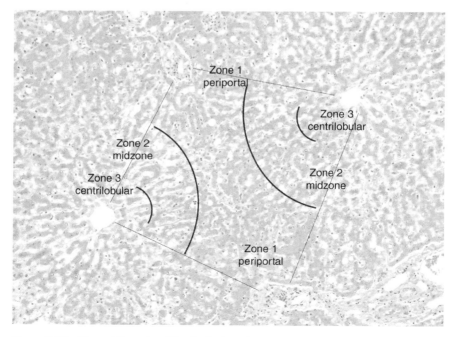

Figure 2.10 Normal liver, dog. Histological section of a Rappaport acinus; notice the black lines that delimit the functional unit (HE, 20×).

blood and consequently, localized damage in this area could be mediated by hypoxic conditions or toxic effects of harmful metabolites (formed as a result of hepatocyte activity in zone 1), as in the detoxification of nonsteroidal antiinflammatory drugs (NSAIDs), reaching the centrilobular area through sinusoidal blood. Finally, there is **zone 2** located between the zones mentioned above (sometimes known as the **midzone**); it is rare for the midzone to be affected alone, but extensive injury starting in the centrilobular region can extend into the midzone.

2.2   Normal Cytology of the Liver

One of the strengths of the diagnostic potential of cytology is the accurate knowledge of normal aspects of the cells that make up either tissue or an anatomical structure. As previously mentioned, only the ability to differentiate the morphological differences of a normal state from the transformations induced by pathological processes creates the necessary conditions to formulate diagnostic criteria, an aspect that is often neglected. In addition to describing the characteristics of the membrane, the cytoplasm (including its content) and the nucleus, the study of cytoarchitecture has recently gained great diagnostic importance. Therefore, the importance of morphological analysis goes well beyond the description of cellular characteristics and also includes the way in which cells tend to organize themselves.

What does normal liver cellularity mean? It refers to the morphological aspects of cells sampled from liver tissue obtained from a clinically healthy patient (with normal levels of liver enzymes and liver function parameters), where ultrasound examination of parenchyma and biliary tract does not show any alterations. While it is true that liver disease can be diagnosed only by comparing clinical, anamnestic, blood and chemistry data, information resulting from ultrasound evaluation of the parenchyma and cytohistological data, unfortunately it is also true that at times in the course of liver disease, the findings resulting from clinical, laboratory, and ultrasound investigations can be perfectly silent. Given the above, I do not actually know how to accurately identify a "truly" healthy patient from which to obtain a representative cytological sample of a normal liver. In the description of the cytological characteristics of a normal liver, I will consequently stick to the findings coming from experience, which are based on observation of the livers of those who are "likely" to be healthy, most of whom have undergone ultrasound-guided sampling, through FNCS performed in order to determine the stage of nonliver-related diseases.

Some cytological alterations that differ from a hypothetical norm of normality are possible even in perfectly healthy livers, so each one of us should formulate a personal concept of cytological normality based on the analysis of as many samples as possible, bearing in mind that even in the presence of minimal morphological characteristics that may suggest pathological processes, a liver may still be considered "normal."

After this necessary caveat, which shows how variable the concept of normality can be within a biological discipline, we will look into everything that can be useful to identify and outline the concept of "normal liver cytology."

2.2.1 Hepatocytes

Cytomorphology: medium-to-large cells, with a diameter of 25–30 μm (3–4 × red blood cell diameter) with a rounded or polygonal shape, indistinct membrane, and finely reticulated cytoplasm that can range, depending on the stain method, from basophilic to eosinophilic [3] (Figures 2.11 and 2.12). There is possible sporadic clearing of the cytoplasm or accumulation of occasional small achromatic globules and the frequent presence of lipofuscin pigment in variable amounts, represented by basophilic granular material dispersed in the cytoplasm (Figure 2.13; see Chapter 3 for a complete description of the appearance and meaning of lipofuscin). Lipofuscin is always present in the cat but can be undetectable in young dogs. There is a round nucleus (slight anisokaryosis should be

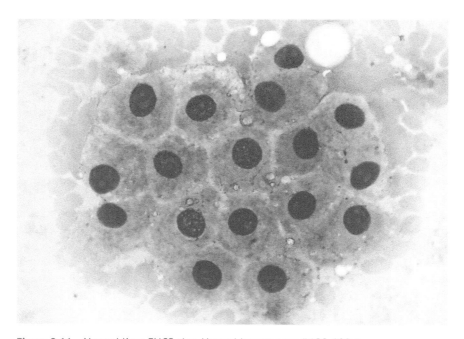

Figure 2.11   Normal liver, FNCS, dog. Normal hepatocytes (MGG, 100×).

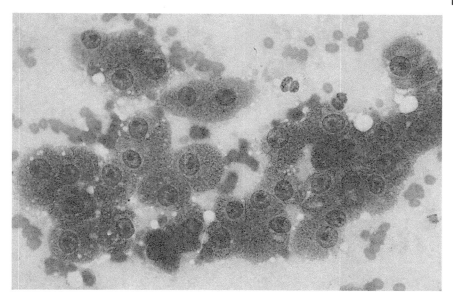

Figure 2.12   Normal liver, FNCS, dog. Normal hepatocytes (Diff-Quik® stain, 40×).

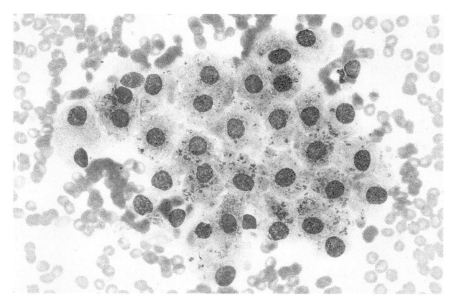

Figure 2.13   Normal liver, FNCS, dog. Normal hepatocytes; in the cytoplasm there is a moderate amount of lipofuscin pigment (MGG, 40×).

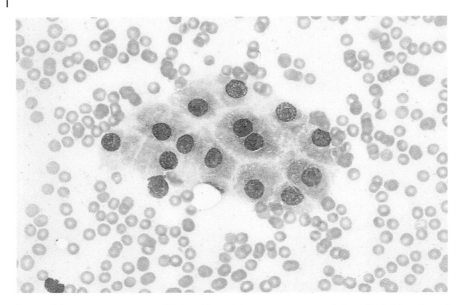

Figure 2.14 Normal liver, FNCS, dog. Normal hepatocytes; one of the cells is binucleated (MGG, 40×).

normal), with finely irregular chromatin; a single nucleolus; double nuclei and more marked anisokaryosis (sometimes indicating regeneration; see Chapter 3 for a description of regenerative changes) are possible, especially in elderly subjects [4] (Figure 2.14). Hepatocytes are distributed in predominantly two-dimensional (sometimes three-dimensional) variably cohesive aggregates, frequently surrounded by smaller groups or single cells; occasionally, cytoplasmic debris and rare naked nuclei can be observed.

Hepatocytes make up the vast majority (80%) of cells found in the liver. FNCS techniques, if carried out in an appropriate manner, always provide hepatocyte-rich samples, so if the samples are poor in hepatocytes – especially when imaging investigations ascertain that the sample comes from the liver – this can be ascribed to sampling errors.

2.2.2 Kupffer Cells

Cytomorphology: small, round, indistinct, lightly basophilic cytoplasm, containing a round and ovoid nucleus with compact chromatin; they are wedged among the hepatocytes and can be identified by their size and nuclear hyperchromatism [5] (Figure 2.15).

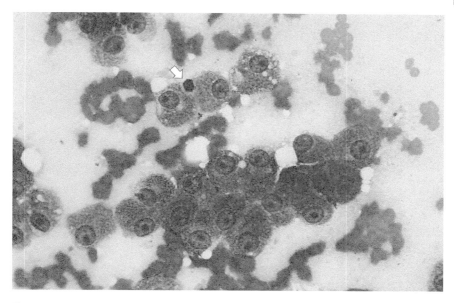

Figure 2.15   Normal liver, FNCS. Kupffer cells (white arrow); notice the small amount of cytoplasm and the dark nucleus (Diff-Quik, 40×).

They represent specialized macrophages localized in the liver; Kupffer cells are the hepatic equivalent of alveolar macrophages in the lung or glia cells in the brain [6]. Detecting and recognizing Kupffer cells in their quiescent form [5] is extremely rare, but it becomes very easy when they are activated due to pathological processes. In this case, they take on a classic rounded shape and become larger, with swelling of the cytoplasm and its contents, which can be ascribed to phagocytosis activity, represented by globular, achromatic or basophilic material; cytophagocytosis is also a feature. The pathological changes will be described in detail in Chapter 6 dedicated to inflammatory processes.

2.2.3   Stellate Cells (Ito Cells)

Cytomorphology: cells with irregularly rounded shape, medium-to-large size (sometimes comparable to a hepatocyte), with dilated cytoplasm due to the presence of achromatic macroglobules; small eccentric nucleus, frequently deformed, with compact chromatin; these cells are wedged individually between the hepatocytes (Figure 2.16).

These are relatively rare cells, located in the space of Disse [7]. Recognizing stellate cells can be difficult as they may be confused with hepatocytes affected by steatosis, which differ in terms of appearance of the nucleus (generally eccentric,

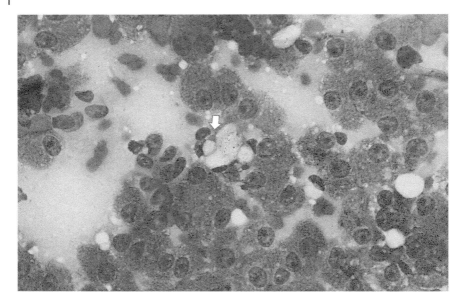

Figure 2.16 Normal liver, FNCS. Stellate (Ito) cells (white arrow): among normal hepatocytes, two cells show cytoplasm filled with achromatic lobules and decentrated nucleus, with dense chromatin (Diff-Quik, 40×).

smaller than that of the hepatocyte and with compact chromatin); the substantial difference is mainly due to the fact that steatosis generally involves quite a number of hepatocytes, while stellate cells exfoliate in a predominantly single form and alternate with relatively normal hepatocytes.

The role of stellate cells is to store vitamin A and, when activated, to contribute to the production of ECM with sinusoidal endotheliocytes. As shown in Chapters 3 and 8 of this book, stellate cells can play a key role in specific pathological processes, such as hyperplastic conditions. They are more abundant in cats than dogs. However, their most relevant role is represented by the potential to transform into myofibroblasts and act as mediators of the deposition of collagen and the progression of liver fibrosis in the course of chronic damage [8].

2.2.4 Cholangiocytes (Biliary Cells)

Cytomorphology: cholangiocytes of the small peripheral ducts include cuboidal, scanty, indistinct and weakly basophilic cytoplasm, as well as a round nucleus with compact chromatin, organized in bidimensional cohesive clusters [3, 9] (Figure 2.17). Cholangiocytes of the large terminal ducts include weakly basophilic columnar cytoplasm and round basal nucleus with granular or compact

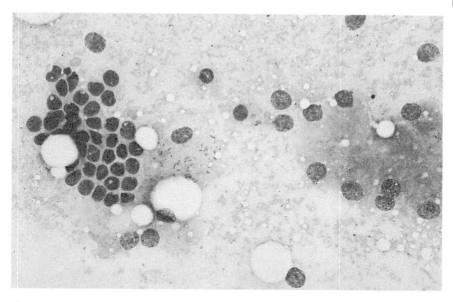

Figure 2.17 Normal liver, FNCS. A small group of normal hepatocytes (to the right) and a cluster of normal biliary cells (to the left). Notice the differences between the two populations: cholangiocytes show indistinct, cuboidal cytoplasm and round to ovoid nucleus, with compact chromatin (MGG, 100×).

chromatin, and are organized in aggregates where palisade arrangements are evident [10] (Figure 2.18).

As in numerous pathological processes, the presence of cholangiocytes in normal liver samples is extremely rare [2]. Therefore, it is most likely a direct consequence of the sampling of parenchymal areas crossed by bile ducts; cholangiocytes are absent in most normal liver samples, although dense clumps of biliary epithelial cells can be observed occasionally [4]. Unlike hepatocytes, which in liver tissue are organized in rows surrounded by sinusoids and consequently easily exfoliate in large numbers, bile ducts of any caliber are generally embedded in the context of the stromal support of the portal space, from which they exfoliate with difficulty and almost always in the course of pathological replication – discussed more in depth in Chapter 9.

2.2.5 Hepatic Lymphocytes

Cytomorphology: small size, scanty basophilic cytoplasm and round nucleus with compact chromatin, individually dispersed.

Resident lymphocytes living in a normal liver are few and virtually indistinguishable from lymphocytes of blood origin. Lymphocytes normally occupy the

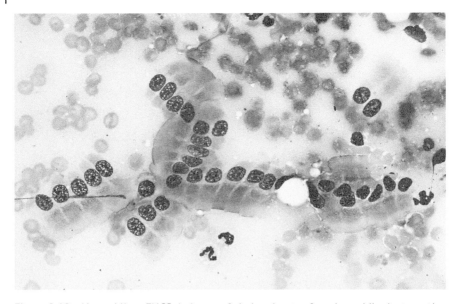

Figure 2.18 Normal liver, FNCS. A cluster of cholangiocytes from large bile ducts; notice the columnar shape and palisading arrangement of the cells (MGG, 40×).

space of Disse and portal triad [11]; they play a key role in immune response. In immunohistochemical studies, T lymphocytes are most abundant [12].

2.2.6 Hepatic Mast Cells

Cytomorphology: small-to-medium size, densely granular cytoplasm, frequently indistinct so as to appear uniformly eosinophilic, round nucleus with irregular or compact chromatin; predominantly single, wedged between hepatocytes or attached to the margins of the aggregates (Figure 2.19).

Mast cells are rare in liver parenchyma and, in dogs, can be found near centrilobular venous vessels [13]; sometimes they are in direct contact with stellate cells [7]. Recognizing them in cytological samples with normal staining techniques can be difficult, but with the application of special, easy-to-use and quick stains, such as toluidine blue (see Chapter 6), their cytoplasmic metachromatic chromatism makes them very easy to identify [14] (Figure 2.20).

2.2.7 Hematopoietic Cells

The liver is a hematopoietic organ during fetal life and hematopoiesis declines after birth, although it continues to occur [15]. In newborn or very

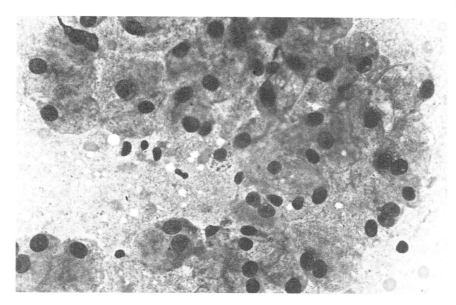

Figure 2.19   Normal liver, FNCS. A single mast cell, with slightly enlarged, granular cytoplasm and round nucleus, located near to a hepatocyte cluster (MGG, 40×).

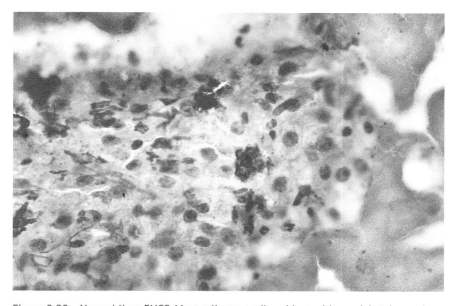

Figure 2.20   Normal liver, FNCS. Mast cells are easily evident with special stains such as toluidine blue (toluidine blue, 40×).

young cats and dogs, under normal conditions, it is possible to observe the presence of hematopoietic elements of the three cell lines: erythroid, myeloid, and thrombocytoid (Figures 2.21 and 2.22).

2.2.8 Mesothelial Cells

Cytomorphology: roundish or polygonal cytoplasm, weakly basophilic, containing a round central nucleus with granular or compact chromatin; organized in pavement-like two-dimensional aggregates, that are sometimes large (Figure 2.23). Mesothelial cells frequently exhibit a pavement-like arrangement with the presence of "windows" seen as intercellular space among the cells and a pink, fuzzy border to the cells [16] (Figure 2.24).

Sampling by needle suction can sometimes result in removal of large sheets of mesothelial elements which delimit the superficial layer of the Glissonian capsule. It is very rare to observe mesothelial cells in liver samples. Generally speaking, their recognition is not difficult as their presence is possible under normal conditions; however, they must not be confused with biliary aggregates, which are rather the result of pathological processes.

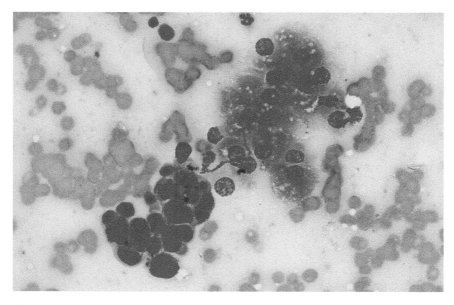

Figure 2.21 Normal liver, FNCS. A cluster of normal hepatocytes and an aggregate of erythroid and myeloid hematopoietic cells (MGG, 100×).

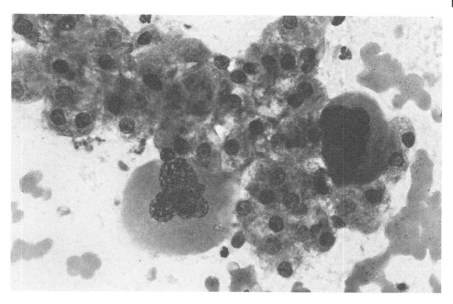

Figure 2.22 Normal liver, FNCS. A cluster of normal hepatocytes and a megakaryocyte (MGG, 100×).

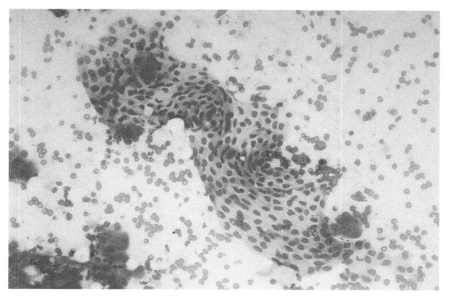

Figure 2.23 Normal liver, FNCS. A single large aggregate of mesothelial cells; notice the distribution in a monodimensional sheet (MGG, 20×).

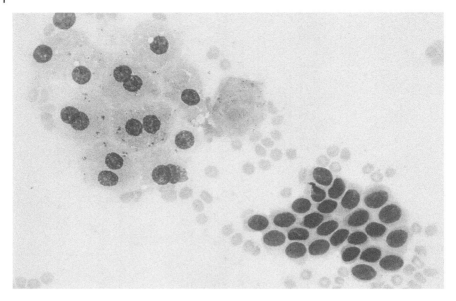

Figure 2.24   Normal liver, FNCS. A cluster of normal hepatocytes (to the left) and a single sheet of mesothelial cells; notice the pink border of the cytoplasm (MGG, 100×).

2.3   Key Points

- Normal hepatocytes may show cytoplasmic accumulation of lipofuscin; moreover, a small amount of blurred or globular achromatic material may be present in some normal hepatocytes.
- Normal cholangiocytes are extremely rarely observed; when present, cholangiopathy must always be suspected and investigated.
- Normal stellate cells, also called Ito cells, exfoliate in low numbers; on the basis of the large, lipid globules inside the cytoplasm, these cells must be differentiated by lipidosis.
- A very small number of lymphocytes may accumulate close to the normal sheets of hepatocytes.
- Normal mast cells exfoliate as single cells, with small cytoplasm, filled with coarse purple granules.
- Mesothelial cells must be differentiated from cholangiocyte sheets.

References

1 Hayes, M.A. (2004). Pathophysiology of the liver. In: *Veterinary Pathophysiology* (ed. R.H. Dunlop and C.H. Malbert), 371–373. Ames, IA: Blackwell Publishing.

2 Rappaport, A.M., Borowy, Z.J., Lougheed, W.M., and Lotto, W.N. (1954). Subdivision of hexagonal liver lobules into a structural and functional unit. Role in hepatic physiology and pathology. *Anat. Rec.* 119 (1): 11–33.

3 Masserdotti, C. (2021). Nonneoplastic disorders of the liver. In: *Veterinary Cytology* (ed. L.C. Sharkey, M.J. Radin, and D. Seelig), 413–416. Hoboken, NJ: Wiley.

4 Stockhaus, C., Teske, E., Van Den Ingh, T. et al. (2002). The influence of age on the cytology of the liver in healthy dogs. *Vet. Pathol.* 39 (1): 154–158.

5 Orell, S.R., Sterret, G.F., Walters, M.N.I. et al. (1992). *Retroperitoneum, Liver and Spleen. Manual and Atlas of Fine Needle Aspiration Cytology*, 247–248. Edinburgh: Churchill Livingstone.

6 Boler, R.K. (1969). Fine structure of canine Kupffer cells and their microtubule-containing cytosomes. *Anat. Rec.* 163 (4): 483–496.

7 Kobayashi, K., Sakata, K., Miyata, K. et al. (1985). Mast cell–Ito cell pairings found in the Disse's spaces in the liver of the beagle dog. *Arch. Histol. Jpn.* 48 (5): 483–496.

8 Ijzer, J., Roskams, T., Molenbeek, R.F. et al. (2006). Morphological characterization of portal myofibroblasts and hepatic stellate cells in the normal dog liver. *Comp. Hepatol.* 16: 5–7.

9 Arndt, T.P. and Shelly, S.M. (2014). The liver. In: *Cowell and Tyler's Diagnostic Cytology of the Dog and Cat*, 4e (ed. A.C. Valenciano and R.L. Cowell), 358–359. St Louis, MO: Elsevier.

10 Meyer, D.K. (2016). The liver. In: *Canine and Feline Cytology – A Color Atlas and Interpretation Guide*, 3e (ed. R.E. Raskin and D.J. Meyer), 259–283. St Louis MO: Elsevier.

11 Sakagami, K., Higaki, K., Toda, K. et al. (1989). Role of canine hepatic sinusoidal lining cells in the immune response. *Transplant. Proc.* 21: 411–415.

12 Weiss, D.J., Gagne, J.M., and Armstrong, P.J. (1989). Characterization of portal lymphocytic infiltrates in feline liver. *Vet. Clin. Pathol.* 21 (1 Pt 1): 411–415.

13 Yamamoto, K. (2000). Electron microscopy of mast cells in the venous wall of canine liver. *J. Vet. Med. Sci.* 62 (11): 1183–1188.

14 Masserdotti, C. (2013). Proportion of mast cells in normal canine hepatic cytologic specimens: comparison of 2 staining methods. *Vet. Clin. Pathol.* 42 (4): 522–525.

15 Crosbie, O.M., Reynolds, M., McEntee, G. et al. (1999). In vitro evidence for the presence of hematopoietic stem cells in the adult human liver. *Hepatology* 29 (4): 1193–1198.

16 Murugan, P., Siddaraju, N., Habeebullah, S., and Basu, D. (2008). Significance of intercellular spaces (windows) in effusion fluid cytology: a study of 46 samples. *Diagn. Cytopathol.* 36 (9): 628–632.

3

Nonspecific and Reversible Hepatocellular Damage

Like cells of other tissues subjected to an insult of some kind, hepatocytes also react to disturbances in their metabolism by manifesting specific morphological alterations, which are mostly characterized by rarefaction and swelling of the cytoplasm.

This range of morphological alterations, which has been called "vacuolar hepatopathy" for a long time [1], is the result of pathological processes that led to a misinterpretation based on a simple morphological survey of the cytoplasmic content; nevertheless, the term is still used and universally accepted for specific lesional processes affecting the hepatocytes. A "vacuole" is a marker of a specific cytoplasmic organelle; furthermore, from an ultrastructural point of view, it is indicative of swelling of a membrane-delimited cytoplasmic structure [2]. The swelling of the cytoplasm appearing during so-called vacuolar hepatopathy is actually a marker of very specific pathological processes determined by the accumulation of achromatic material, which, from an ultrastructural point of view, never remains within a membrane-delimited structure, as it disperses in the cytoplasm [3, 4].

On the base of these considerations, the use of the terms "vacuole" and "vacuolar" is, in my opinion, not correct and should be discontinued in scientific literature. In addition, the achromatic material that swells the cytoplasm (sometimes recognizable using special stains) can be of a very different nature and correspond to independent pathological processes. The term "vacuolar hepatopathy" may lead to a generalization of the pathogenesis, resulting in loss of morphological meaning and, consequently, disregard of potential associations with certain primary causes. In light of the above, it would be appropriate to replace the term "vacuolar liver disease" with "rarefaction of the cytoplasm" or, better, "nonspecific reversible hepatocellular damage" which, aside from being recognized by the WSAVA standard, is equally nonspecific but more indicative of the alterations that will be discussed in this chapter. Personally, in my reports, I use the term "nonspecific reversible hepatocellular damage" when I describe alterations whose

Canine and Feline Liver Cytology, First Edition. Carlo Masserdotti.
© 2024 John Wiley & Sons, Inc. Published 2024 by John Wiley & Sons, Inc.

comparison with clinical and anamnestic data, as well as with laboratory diagnostics or diagnostic imaging, suggests a potentially curable liver disease. Whenever I observe the same alterations but with accessory and secondary significance – associated with morphological data that indicate a progressive and irreversible process (such as the presence of fibrosis or either hyperplastic or neoplastic phenomena) – I only use the term "nonspecific hepatocellular damage."

Reversible and nonspecific damage of hepatocytes is associated with swelling of the cytoplasm with formation of membrane-surrounded blebs of cytoplasm, which protrude and consequently alter the profile of the cell itself. This phenomenon is mediated by damage to the cytoskeleton, induced by the disruption of Ca^{++} ions homeostasis. This phenomenon (also called "blebbing," see Chapter 1) includes the formation and detachment from the intact cell of vesicles containing hepatocytic enzymes [5]; when the blebs enter the bloodstream, after their dissolution, the enzymes they contain, such ALT or AST, are delivered; this leads to increased levels of hepatic enzymes in blood, as occurs in many hepatopathies. The concentration of these enzymes can be variable but it generally increases when the damage to the hepatocytes is more severe and extensive, although without a real quantitative correlation with the extent of damage. For this reason, it is not possible to correlate specific cellular damage (even in cases of very high concentration of liver enzymes), without the necessary morphological investigations.

What does "reversible nonspecific hepatocellular damage" mean? Generally speaking, it means a state of cytoplasmic insult determined by the accumulation of achromatic material, whose causes are generally very common, diverse and thus hard to identify ("nonspecific") from a diagnostic point of view. If the pathological cause is resolved, the hepatocytes tend to return to their original structural and morphological integrity ("reversible") [6]. The ability to recognize a specific type of material accumulated in the cytoplasm aids in diagnosis of differential causes.

As discussed in Chapter 12 on nodular lesions of the hepatic parenchyma, the same nonspecific damage is also frequently detected in samples of hyperplastic nodular lesions, as well as during neoplastic transformation; in these cases, the accumulation cannot be considered "reversible" due to the hyperplastic or neoplastic nature of the process. This hepatocellular damage can be caused by the vascular alterations that often occur at the onset of nodular lesions – presumably as a consequence of disturbances affecting the normal supply of oxygen and nutritional substances.

3.1 Accumulation of Water

Cytomorphology: roundish or polygonal hepatocyte cytoplasm, increased size, loss of normal reticulated texture and bluish color, due to accumulation of dispersed achromatic material (Figure 3.1); round nucleus with irregular chromatin (sometimes with a single nucleolus); possible rupture of some hepatocytes.

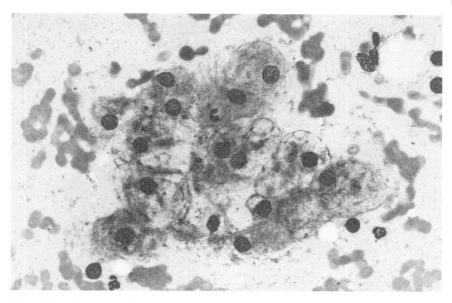

Figure 3.1 Liver, reversible hepatic injury, FNCS, dog. Hepatocytes are enlarged and the cytoplasm is filled with achromatic material; without special stains, it is not morphologically possible to differentiate water from glycogen accumulation (MGG, 100×).

Hydropic change is a marker of almost every form of hepatocellular damage, especially in the initial stages; it has also been defined in the literature as "cloudy swelling" or "hydropic degeneration" [6]. This is a consequence of the inability to maintain homeostasis of ionic exchanges and cytoplasmic water. In terms of morphology, hepatocytes swell (accumulation of achromatic material with blurred edges), losing their typical finely reticulated texture and the basophilic color of the cytoplasm. Morphologically, it is impossible to differentiate this hepatocellular damage from the accumulation of intracytoplasmic glycogen (discussed below); therefore, in those very rare cases in which this distinction is necessary, special stains such as periodic acid-Schiff (PAS) may be useful, since accumulation of water is negative with this stain.

3.2   Accumulation of Glycogen

Cytomorphology: rounded or polygonal cytoplasm, increased dimensions (sometimes considerable), loss of normal reticulated texture and bluish color due to rarefaction caused by the accumulation of dispersed achromatic material (Figures 3.2 and 3.3); round nucleus with irregular chromatin; in cases of considerable swelling, the cytoplasmic profile may feature sharp margins (Figure 3.4); possible rupture of some hepatocytes.

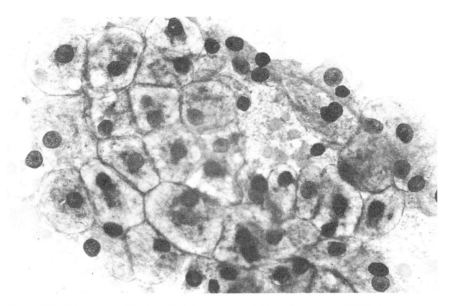

Figure 3.2 Liver, reversible hepatic injury, accumulation of glycogen, FNCS, dog. Hepatocytes are enlarged and the cytoplasm is filled with a large amount of achromatic material; distinction between water and glycogen accumulation is not morphologically possible (MGG, 100×).

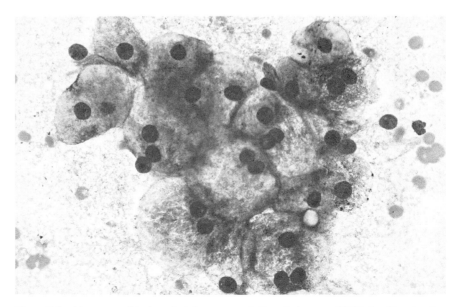

Figure 3.3 Liver, reversible hepatic injury, accumulation of glycogen, FNCS, dog. Hepatocytes are enlarged and the cytoplasm is filled with achromatic material; notice that with a different Romanowsky-modified stain, although the color of the cells is different compared with cells in Figure 3.2, the achromatic material has similar features (Diff-Quik® stain, 100×).

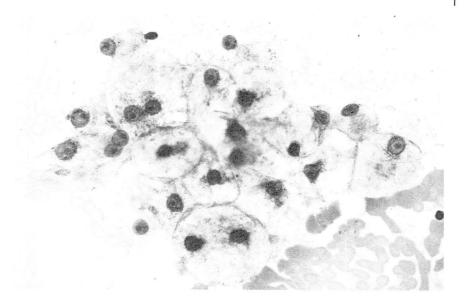

Figure 3.4 Liver, reversible hepatic injury, accumulation of glycogen, FNCS, dog. Note the sharp border of enlarged cells with accumulation of cytoplasmic achromatic material (MGG, 100×).

The characteristic cytoplasmic accumulation of glycogen occurs when induced by endogenous or exogenous corticosteroids and has always been referred to as "steroid-induced liver disease" [7, 8] (Figure 3.5). This cytoplasmic change tends to be associated with conditions that cause an increase in adrenal secretion of cortisol. Excess cortisol can be the result of endocrine diseases affecting the pituitary or adrenal glands or iatrogenic administration of corticosteroid drugs. However, almost any chronic stressful pathological event can induce the adrenal gland to produce cortisol, which widens the spectrum of possible causes to a virtually endless list of chronic extrahepatic diseases, such as renal, immune-mediated, cardiac, hepatobiliary, neoplastic, neurological, and gastrointestinal conditions [1] (Table 3.1).

From a morphological point of view, swelling of the hepatocyte cytoplasm is due to accumulation of achromatic material with blurred edges (comparable to what is normally observed during water accumulation); in addition, it may double in size and, in extreme cases, the peripheral cytoplasmic profile appears as if it had been drawn with a pencil (Figure 3.6). I personally do not believe that distinguishing these two conditions is clinically useful, but whenever necessary (rarely), the accumulation of glycogen can be effectively demonstrated through the use of PAS staining (Figure 3.7) and diastase. PAS detects polysaccharides such as glycogen, glycoprotein, glycolipids, and mucins; glycogen appears deep purple with PAS and achromatic after the action of diastase, which breaks down glycogen.

(a)   (b)

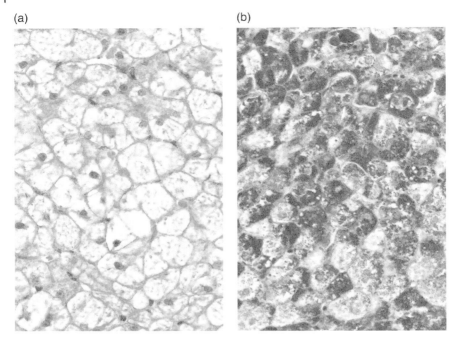

Figure 3.5   Liver, accumulation of glycogen, dog. Enlarged hepatocytes look like the cells in cytology samples; compare the section of liver stained with HE (a) and with PAS (b) (HE, PAS, 40×).

3.3   Accumulation of Lipids

Cytomorphology: roundish or polygonal shape of the cytoplasm, that appears increased in size; loss of typical fine reticulated texture and bluish color due to accumulation of achromatic material represented by achromatic globules with sharply demarcated margins that sometimes push the nuclei to the periphery of the cytoplasm (Figures 3.8 and 3.9). Macrovesicular steatosis features globules with a diameter similar to or greater than that of the nucleus, sometimes in low numbers or even single (Figure 3.10); profile of the globules frequently overlaps the outline of the nucleus (Figure 3.11). In microvesicular steatosis lipidic globules are even smaller than the nucleus and tend to overlap the nuclear profile (Figures 3.12 and 3.13). Lipids without and outside the cytoplasm may be oxidized, as a consequence of artifacts that occur after sampling, and appear as eosinophilic globules (Figure 3.14). The cytoplasm may contain small granules of lipofuscin (Figure 3.15); extracytoplasmic cholestasis may be observed, as small casts of biliary material among the cells (Figure 3.16).

Table 3.1   Percentage of underlying diseases identified in dogs with glycogen accumulation.

Underlying disease	Percentage
Renal disease	3.6
Chronic renal disease	2.1
Glomerulonephritis	0.6
Other	0.9
Immune-mediated disease	10.1
Hemolytic anemia	3.6
Thrombocytopenia	1.8
Hemolytic anemia and thrombocytopenia	1.8
Systemic lupus erythematosus	1.2
Other	1.8
Cardiac disease	1.5
Congestive heart failure	0.9
Other	0.6
Acquired hepatobiliary disease	12.8
Chronic hepatitis, cirrhosis, liver failure	3.3
Cholangiohepatitis or cholangitis	2.4
Hepatotoxicosis	1.5
Hepatic fibrosis	1.2
Cholecystitis	1.2
Extrahepatic bile duct obstruction	0.9
Hepatocutaneous syndrome	0.9
Acute liver failure	0.9
Other	0.9
Adrenal gland disfunction	11.9
Pituitary-dependent hyperadrenocorticism	6.3
Adrenal neoplasia	4.2
Sex hormone adrenal hyperplasia	0.9
Other	0.6
Neoplasia	28
Lymphoma	5.7
Adenocarcinoma	4.5
Hemangiosarcoma	3.9

(Continued)

Table 3.1 (Continued)

Underlying disease	Percentage
Meningioma	1.5
Leukemia	1.2
Multiple tumors	1.2
Hepatoma	1.2
Transitional cell carcinoma	0.9
Osteosarcoma	0.9
Hepatocellular carcinoma	0.9
Pheochromocytoma	0.9
Other	5.4
Neurological disease	11.3
Intervertebral disc disease	2.1
Degenerative myelopathy	2.4
Wobbler syndrome	0.9
Peripheral neuropathy	0.9
Other	5.1
Gastrointestinal tract disease	9.2
Inflammatory bowel disease	3.6
Pancreatitis	2.4
Pancreatitis and inflammatory bowel disease	0.9
Peritonitis	0.9
Other	1.5
Portosystemic vascular anomaly	3.9
Infectious disease	1.8
Diabetes mellitus	0.9
Miscellaneous	5.1

Source: Adapted from Sepesey et al. 2006 [1].

This type of damage consists of cytoplasmic accumulation of lipids. As in several other cytological events, lipids are present in the form of achromatic globules with rounded profile and sharp margins. In the literature, this has been defined in various ways, including "steatosis" (accumulation of triglycerides) and "lipidosis" (generic accumulation of lipids). However, despite the difference between the two terms [9], they are used interchangeably. The causes are numerous and range

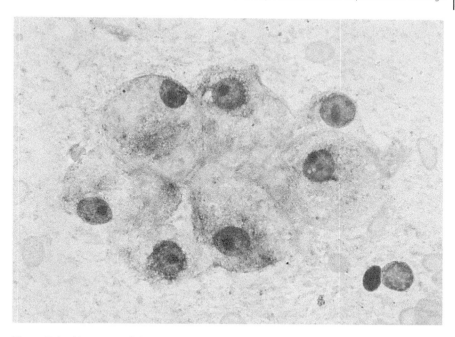

Figure 3.6 Liver, reversible hepatic injury, accumulation of glycogen, FNCS, dog.
Extremely enlarged cytoplasm with sharp borders (MGG, 100×).

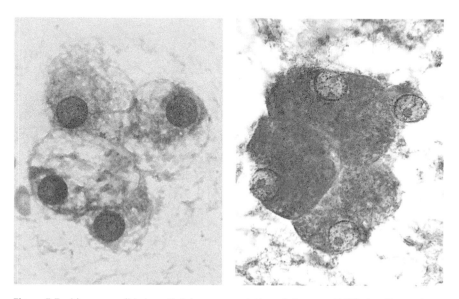

Figure 3.7 Liver, reversible hepatic injury, accumulation of glycogen, FNCS, dog. Comparison
of glycogen accumulation, represented by achromatic material with Romanwsky-modified
stains to the left and deep purple with PAS to the right (MGG, PAS, 100×).

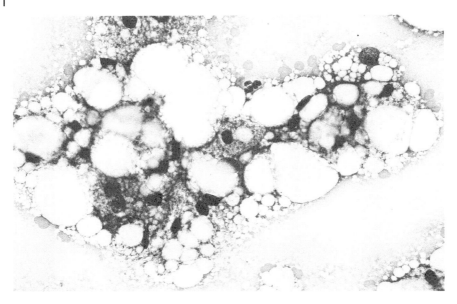

Figure 3.8 Liver, reversible hepatic injury, steatosis, FNCS, cat. Cells are enlarged and the cytoplasm is filled with achromatic globules with sharp margins that sometimes push the nuclei to the periphery (MGG, 100×).

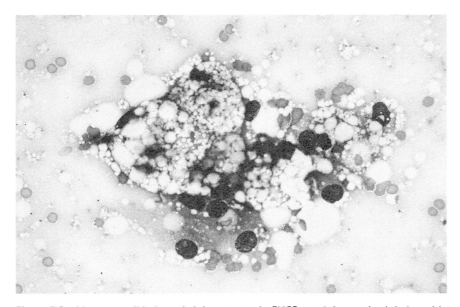

Figure 3.9 Liver, reversible hepatic injury, steatosis, FNCS, cat. Achromatic globules with sharp margin; notice the different size of the globules and the nuclei pushed to the periphery (MGG, 100×).

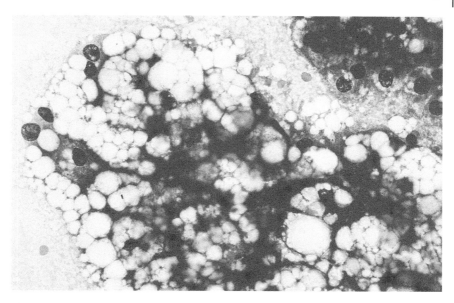

Figure 3.10 Liver, reversible hepatic injury, steatosis, FNCS, cat. In macrovesicular steatosis, the size of lipid droplets is greater than the diameter of the nucleus (MGG, 100×).

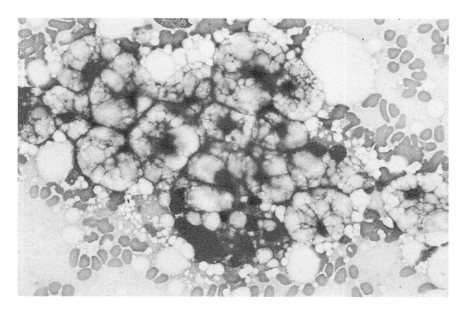

Figure 3.11 Liver, reversible hepatic injury, steatosis, FNCS, cat. Sometimes the lipid globules overlap the profile of the nucleus (MGG, 100×).

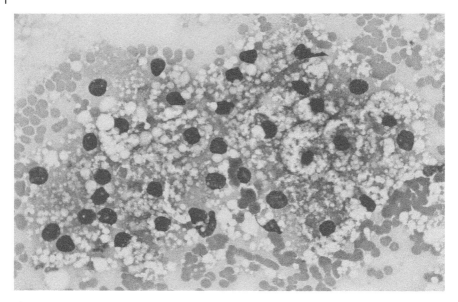

Figure 3.12 Liver, reversible hepatic injury, steatosis, FNCS, cat. In microvesicular steatosis, the size of the lipid globules is smaller than the diameter of the nucleus (MGG, 100×).

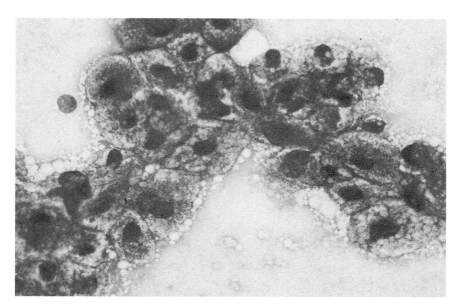

Figure 3.13 Liver, reversible hepatic injury, steatosis, FNCS, dog. In microvesicular steatosis, the sharp outline of small globules helps in distinction from glycogen accumulation (MGG, 100×).

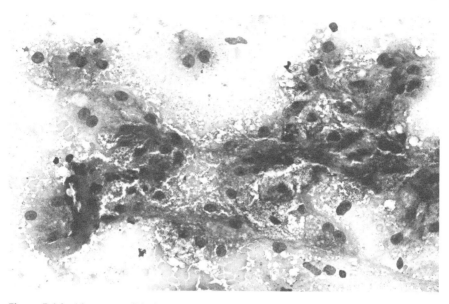

Figure 3.14 Liver, reversible hepatic injury, steatosis, FNCS, dog The hepatocytes are filled with fat globules; notice the presence of small aggregates of yellow-brown material in some cells, recognizable as oxidized fat (MGG, 100×).

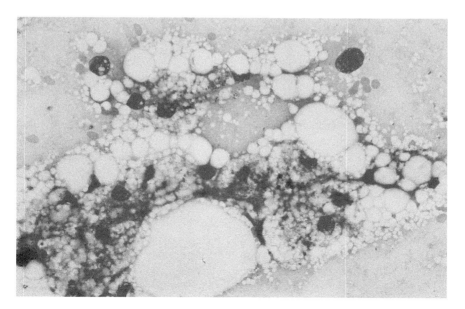

Figure 3.15 Liver, reversible hepatic injury, steatosis, FNCS, dog. Notice the presence of small aggregates of bluish material, recognizable as lipofuscin, inside the cytoplasm together with fat globules (MGG, 100×).

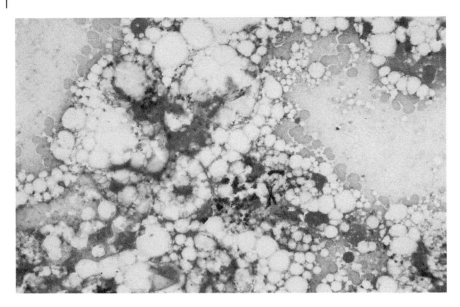

Figure 3.16 Liver, reversible hepatic injury, steatosis, FNCS, cat. Among the cytoplasm of these cells filled with fat globules, there are casts of biliary material (MGG, 100×).

from conditions that determine a higher influx of lipids due to increased dietary intake or increased mobilization of adipose tissue, to decreased metabolizing ability of the hepatocytic cytoplasmic systems or decreased ability to export lipoproteins in the posthepatic capillary stream. The hepatocytes affected by steatosis exfoliate and deposit on a background that is generally cluttered with abundant achromatic globular material – depending on how many of them underwent breakdown during set-up operations.

In the course of "macrovesicular steatosis," the globules containing lipid material that accumulate in the cytoplasm are larger than those contained in the nucleus, which normally results in swelling of the cytoplasm and displacement of the nucleus in the periphery. In contrast, in "microvesicular steatosis" the globules are smaller than the nucleus, to the point that their globular appearance may be difficult to recognize (especially in the absence of displacement); in addition, in some extreme cases, they may even overlap the profile of the nucleus. From a morphological point of view, micro- and macrovesicular steatosis, a mix of the two types, is not particularly difficult to recognize, as the findings are very peculiar, especially when this phenomenon involves all the hepatocytes.

In cases where it is difficult to determine if microvesicular steatosis is caused by glycogen or water accumulation, oil red O staining of unfixed slides can be used to confirm lipid accumulation [10]. Using an air-dried slide, place one drop of oil red O and, after few minutes, counterstain it with new methylene blue; the lipidic globules in the cytoplasm will appear bright orange (Figure 3.17).

Although the recognition of lipids is generally easy, attempting to establish the causes of steatosis and distinguishing between micro- and macrovesicular steatosis are particularly difficult. Although this is not the ideal place to fully discuss the key role of the liver in lipid metabolism, a list of the causes of steatosis includes the following:

- excessive influx of lipids from the diet
- increased mobilization of lipids from adipose tissue
- reduced availability of energy for the oxidation of fatty acids (hypoxia)
- toxic mitochondrial damage with alteration of beta-oxidation
- increased esterification of fatty acids to triglycerides, induced by an increase in glucose or insulin (hyperadrenocorticism)
- decreased lipoprotein synthesis (dietary deficiencies, toxins or adverse drug reactions)
- decreased secretory export of lipoproteins (toxins or adverse drug reactions).

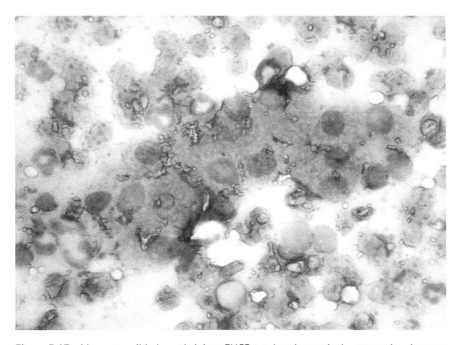

Figure 3.17 Liver, reversible hepatic injury, FNCS, cat. In microvesicular steatosis, whenever necessary, oil red O stains lipidic material that appears bright orange (oil red O, 100×).

In human pathology, the literature on the subject is vast, while in veterinary medicine there are well-known associations between diabetes and microvesicular steatosis in dogs [11] or microvesicular steatosis and juvenile hypoglycemia [12]. In cats, steatosis with a mixed micro- and macrovesicular appearance is typically found in the so-called feline idiopathic lipidosis [9]. The cytological diagnosis of this condition is possible when at least 80% of the hepatocytes are affected by the alteration (Figure 3.18), preferably if combined with specific anamnestic results, blood chemistry, and ultrasonographic investigations [13, 14]. The pathogenesis normally includes an energetic imbalance caused by periods of anorexia, generally induced by primary diseases; furthermore, obesity is also considered a predisposing risk factor. Hematochemical investigations may show an increase in the concentration of liver enzymes, as well as a decrease in the concentration of urea, albumin, and possibly hyperglycemia. Heinz bodies in circulating erythrocytes may be detected, a marker of oxidative damage [13]. Nevertheless, these alterations are generally caused by primary diseases.

(a)   (b)

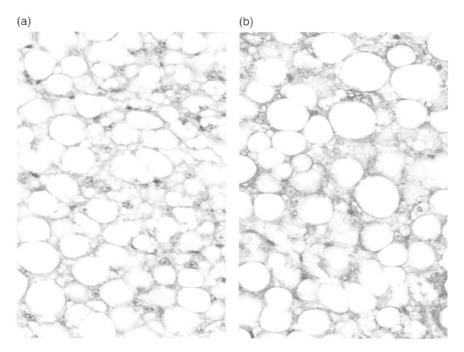

Figure 3.18 Liver, hepatic steatosis, cat. Large globules of fat enlarge the cytoplasm of the hepatocytes (a), similar to cytological samples. (b) Notice that cytoplasmic content is negative with PAS stain (HE, PAS, 40×).

A very rare cause of microvesicular lipidosis in young cats is lysosomal storage disease, such as Niemann–Pick disease type C [15].

I believe that steatosis is probably the most difficult nonspecific and reversible damage to interpret and, consequently, reliable considerations about the causes are not possible without comparison with all the clinical and anamnestic data, as well as with those from laboratory diagnostics. As aspecific change, steatosis seems to be, in my experience, very frequent in cats as consequence of many primary causes, while in dogs it is rare.

3.4 Accumulation of Bilirubin and Bile Salts

Cytomorphology: rounded or polygonal hepatocyte cytoplasm, increased size (sometimes considerable), loss of normal reticulated texture and bluish color due to accumulation of dispersed achromatic material; round nucleus with irregular chromatin on which the described material often deposits; no specific way to differentiate the accumulation of water from that of glycogen.

This type of hepatocellular damage is described by the WSAVA standard as intracytoplasmic cholestasis and defined as "feathery degeneration" [16], which cannot be cytomorphologically recognized. The accumulation of bilirubin and intracytoplasmic bile salts is detectable via electron microscopy, but it appears similar to the accumulation of glycogen or water. It is important to emphasize that the cytoplasmic accumulation of bilirubin is morphologically impossible to recognize and that this condition is very different from the accumulation of extracytoplasmic bilirubin, which, as discussed in Chapter 4, includes specific features that are very easy to detect represented by linear or branched casts of biliary material, accumulated among the cytoplasm of the hepatocytes.

3.5 Hyperplasia of Stellate Cells

Cytomorphology: presence of an increased number of round cells with large achromatic globules, mostly single, that displace the round to ovoid nucleus at the periphery; these cells are located among normal or slightly injured hepatocytes (Figure 3.19).

The hyperplasia of stellate cells may be confused with hepatic lipidosis. To differentiate the two conditions, always bear in mind that stellate cells show enlarged, globular cytoplasm and are scattered among almost normal hepatocytes, while in steatosis a variable amount of lipidic globule accumulation is always evident inside the cytoplasm of hepatocytes. Although not directly

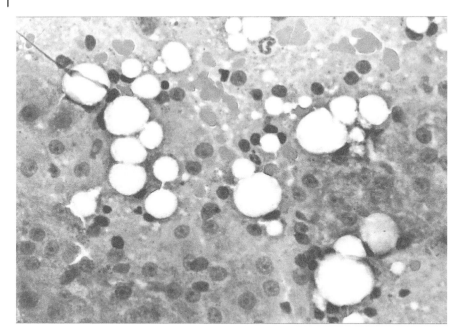

Figure 3.19 Liver, stellate cell hyperplasia, FNCS, cat. In this aggregate of hepatocytes, there are some cells with round, indistinct cytoplasm, filled with large globules that displace the nucleus to the periphery (MGG, 40×).

related to hepatocellular change, this chapter seems to be the right place to discuss the topic. Normal stellate cells, also known as "Ito cells," located in the space of Disse show an irregularly roundish shape and are present in very low numbers among the hepatocytes. In their resting state, they store vitamin A, represented as lipidic vitamin, in large unstained droplets; when activated by chronic injury, they are involved in the processes that lead to fibrosis. Other than transformation to myofibroblasts during chronic injury changes, a pathological condition observed mostly in old cats, but sometimes in old dogs, is well known [17]. This change is represented by an increased number of stellate cells, with an enlarged cytoplasm filled with large globules that displace the nucleus to the periphery. Etiological causes are not well understood, although senile changes are suspected.

Chronic vitamin A intoxication has been described in cats fed with raw beef liver, with hyperplasia and hypertrophy of stellate cells, liver fibrosism and bone esostoses [18]. The diagnostic key to distinguish these changes from hepatic lipidosis is comparison of the increased number of enlarged stellate cells with normal hepatocytes (Figure 3.20).

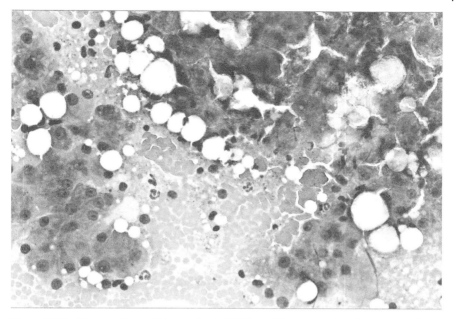

Figure 3.20   Liver, stellate cell hyperplasia, FNCS, cat. The comparison between stellate cells, which show globular cytoplasm, and hepatocytes, which are almost normal, is helpful in distinguishing between steatosis and Ito cell hyperplasia (MGG, 40×).

3.6   Regenerative Changes

Cytomorphology: the cytoplasm of hepatocytes looks almost normal, although a variable degree of reversible change may be observed (Figure 3.21); difference in size of hepatocytes is frequently observed; anisokaryosis is generally mild to moderate but abnormal nuclei may be detected (Figures 3.22 and 3.23); binucleated cells are frequently seen (Figure 3.24); trinucleated cells, although rare, may be observed (Figure 3.25); chromatin is generally irregularly granular, nucleoli are small; mytosis of mature hepatocytes is an occasional finding (Figure 3.26); possible to observe regenerative changes together with inflammation or fibrosis (Figure 3.27).

Although regeneration is not considered a "reversible nonspecific change," we discuss it in this chapter since the features are nonspecific and detectable in many pathological conditions. Regeneration refers to the ability of the liver to ensure that the liver-to-body weight ratio is always at 100% of what is required for body homeostasis; experimental models that involve partial hepatectomy or chemical injury have revealed extracellular and intracellular signaling pathways

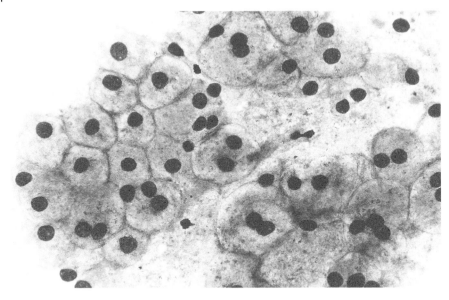

Figure 3.21 Liver, hepatocellular regeneration, FNCS, dog. Regenerative hepatocytes show variable degrees of reversible change, as accumulation of water or glycogen (MGG, 100×).

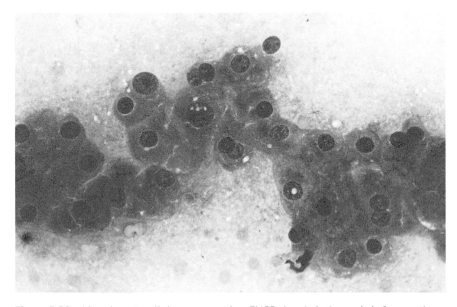

Figure 3.22 Liver, hepatocellular regeneration, FNCS, dog. Anisokaryosis is frequently evident (MGG, 100×).

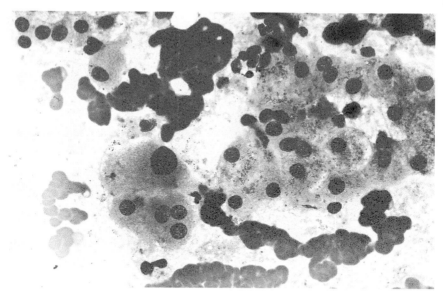

Figure 3.23 Liver, hepatocellular regeneration, FNCS, dog. Large, abnormal nuclei are sometimes evident (MGG, 100×).

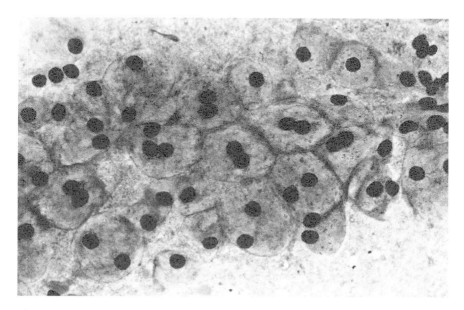

Figure 3.24 Liver, hepatocellular regeneration, FNCS, dog. Many cells are binucleated, and sometimes trinucleated (MGG, 100×).

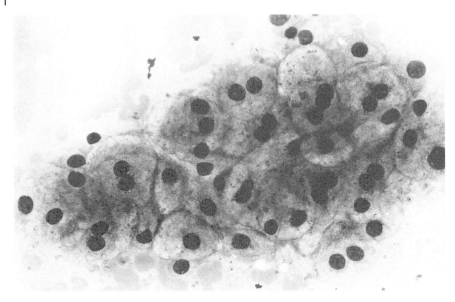

Figure 3.25 Liver, hepatocellular regeneration, FNCS, dog. Binucleated and trinucleated cells (MGG, 100×).

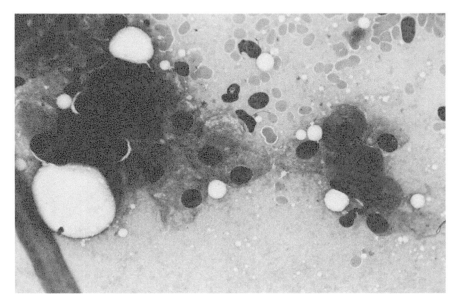

Figure 3.26 Liver, hepatocellular regeneration, FNCS, dog. Mitotic figures, although rare, should be considered as regenerative change when observed in aggregates of mature hepatocytes (MGG, 100×).

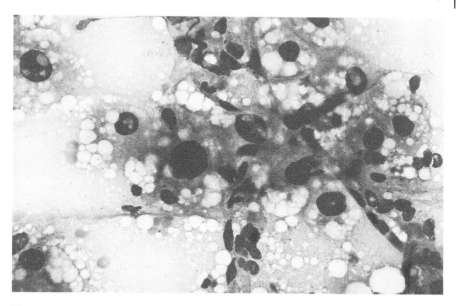

Figure 3.27 Liver, hepatocellular regeneration, FNCS, dog. Regenerative changes may be observed together with signs of chronic damage, such as fibrosis (MGG, 100×).

that are used to return the liver to equivalent size and weight to those prior to injury [19]. Regeneration involves not only the stem progenitor cells but also the mature hepatocytes, which may proliferate to restore the damaged cells [19]. Injury or loss of hepatocytes, which can occur in acute or chronic liver disease of any etiology, including inflammation, fibrosis, and cirrhosis, may induce regeneration, cytologically represented by the described features, although it may also be age related. The most evident change is represented by binucleated, occasionally trinucleated hepatocytes, with a mild to moderate degree of anisokaryosis and anisocytosis [20]. Care must be taken in evaluation of mild to moderate anisokaryosis, when nonnodular liver is investigated, in order to avoid an incorrect diagnosis of malignancy. The difference from hepatocellular carcinoma (see Chapter 12) is mostly represented by a clinical description of a hepatic mass and, from the cytological point of view, by the presence of naked nuclei crowded around hepatocytes. In rare cases of poorly differentiated hepatocellular carcinoma, anisokaryosis may be severe, together with clumped chromatin and large nucleoli, while in regeneration chromatin is generally granular and nucleoli are small.

Regenerative changes require future studies in order to be better understood.

3.7 Key Points

- Aspecific reversible changes may be the consequence of well-known causes, such as glycogen accumulation induced by steroid or lipid accumulation induced by diabetes. Nevertheless, accumulation of water, glycogen or lipids are aspecific changes that may be a consequence of many primary causes, in most instances not recognizable. Glycogen accumulation is much more evident in dogs, while steatosis is evident mostly in cats.
- Accumulation of glycogen is not distinguishable from accumulation of water, although accumulation of glycogen, mostly in dogs, is much more frequent than accumulation of water. To differentiate the two conditions, when necessary, the use of special stains such as PAS and PAS with diastase is necessary.
- Distinguishing microvesicular from macrovesicular steatosis should help in recognition of different causes.
- Accumulation of intracytoplasmic bilirubin and bile salts is indicated by aspecific changes that are not distinguishable as water or glycogen accumulation.
- Hyperplasia of stellate cells, described in the cat, is suggested by the presence of round cells with enlarged cytoplasm, filled with achromatic, lipid globules scattered among normal or slightly injured hepatocytes.
- Care must be taken when in samples from nonnodular liver hepatocytes are featured by anisocytosis and anisokaryosis; this must be interpreted mostly as regeneration of hepatocytes, that occurs after injury or is age related.

References

1 Sepesy, L.M., Center, S.A., Randolph, J.F. et al. (2006). Vacuolar hepatopathy in dogs: 336 cases (1993–2005). *J. Am. Vet. Med. Assoc.* 229 (2): 246–252.
2 Bloom, W. and Fawcett, D.W. (1981). The cell and cell division. In: *A Textbook of Histology* (ed. W. Bloom and D.W. Fawcett), 48–51. Padua: Piccin Editore.
3 Rutgers, H.C., Batt, R.M., Vaillant, C., and Riley, J.E. (1995). Subcellular pathologic features of glucocorticoid-induced hepatopathy in dogs. *Am. J. Vet. Res.* 56 (7): 898–907.
4 DiAugustine, R.P., Schaefer, J.M., and Fouts, J.R. (1973). Hepatic lipid droplets. Isolation, morphology and composition. *Biochem. J.* 132 (2): 323–327.
5 Cullen, J.M. (2005). Mechanistic classification of liver injury. *Toxicol. Pathol.* 33 (1): 6–8.
6 Cullen, J.M., van den Ingh, T.S.G.A.M., van Winkle, T. et al. (2006). Morphological classification of parenchymal disorders of the canine and feline liver – normal histology, reversible hepatocytic injury and hepatic amyloidosis. In: *Standard for Clinical and Histological Diagnosis of Canine and Feline Liver Disease* (ed. WSAVA Liver Standardization Group), 77–79. St Louis, MO: Saunders.

7 Schaer, M. and Ginn, P.E. (1999). Iatrogenic Cushing's syndrome and steroid hepatopathy in a cat. *J. Am. Anim. Hosp. Assoc.* 35 (1): 48–51.

8 Kuhlenschmidt, M.S., Hoffmann, W.E., and Rippy, M.K. (1991). Glucocorticoid hepatopathy: effect on receptor-mediated endocytosis of asialoglycoproteins. *Biochem. Med. Metab. Biol.* 46 (2): 152–168.

9 Cullen, J.M., van den Ingh, T.S.G.A.M., van Winkle, T. et al. (2006). Morphological classification of parenchymal disorders of the canine and feline liver – normal histology, reversible hepatocytic injury and hepatic amyloidosis. In: *Standard for Clinical and Histological Diagnosis of Canine and Feline Liver Disease* (ed. WSAVA Liver Standardization Group), 80–82. St Louis, MO: Saunders.

10 Masserdotti, C., Bonfanti, U., de Lorenzi, D. (2004). Oil Red O in cytologic samples of feline hepatic lipidosis. *Proceedings of 6th Annual ESVCP Meeting with 22th ESVP Congress* (15–18 September 2004), Olsztyn, Poland.

11 Lettow, E. and Lopponow, H. (1972). Funktionelle und morphologische Untersuchungen der Leber bei Hunden mit manifestem und latentem Diabetes mellitus. *Proceedings of the Gaines European Veterinary Symposium, Amsterdam. Gaines*, 25–28 March, 1972.

12 Van del Linde-Sipman, J.S., van den Ingh, T.S.G.A.M., and van Toor, A.J. Fatty liver syndrome in puppies. *J. Am. Anim. Hosp. Assoc.* 13 (1): 16–23.

13 Kuzi, S., Segev, G., Kedar, S. et al. (2017). Prognostic markers in feline hepatic lipidosis: a retrospective study of 71 cats. *Vet. Rec.* 181 (19): 512.

14 Valtolina, C. and Favier, R.P. (2017). Feline hepatic lipidosis. *Vet. Clin. Small Anim. Pract.* 47 (3): 683–702.

15 Brown, D.E., Thrall, M.A., Walkley, S.U. et al. (1994). Feline Niemann–Pick disease type C. *Am. J. Pathol.* 144 (6): 1412–1415.

16 Cullen, J.M., van den Ingh, T.S.G.A.M., van Winkle, T. et al. (2006). Morphological classification of parenchymal disorders of the canine and feline liver: 1. Normal histology, reversible hepatocytic injury and hepatic amyloidosis. In: *Standard for Clinical and Histological Diagnosis of Canine and Feline Liver Disease* (ed. WSAVA Liver Standardization Group), 79–80. St Louis, MO: Saunders.

17 Van Winkle, T., Cullen, J.M., van den Ingh, T.S.G.A.M. et al. (2006). Morphological classification of parenchymal disorders of the canine and feline liver: 3. Hepatic abscesses and granulomas, hepatic metabolic storage disorders and miscellaneous conditions. In: *Standard for Clinical and Histological Diagnosis of Canine and Feline Liver Disease* (ed. WSAVA Liver Standardization Group), 103–116. St. Louis, MO: Saunders.

18 Guerra, J.M., Daniel, A.G.T., Aloia, T.P.A. et al. (2014). Hypervitaminosis A-induced hepatic fibrosis in a cat. *J. Feline Med. Surg.* 16 (3): 243–248.

19 Michalopoulos, G.K. and Bhushan, B. (2021). Liver regeneration: biological and pathological mechanisms and implications. *Nat. Rev. Gastroenterol. Hepatol.* 18 (1): 40–55.

20 Koss, L.G., Woyke, S., and Olszewski, W. (1992). The liver. In: *Aspiration Biopsy: Cytologic Interpretation and Histologic Bases*. Tokyo, Japan: Igaku-Shoin.

4

Intracytoplasmic and Extracytoplasmic Pathological Accumulation

As discussed in the previous chapter, morphological alterations affecting the hepatocyte include abnormal accumulations of achromatic material, a marker of nonspecific and reversible damage, which by definition tends to resolve when primary damage disappears. Other substances can accumulate in the cytoplasm due to pathological processes (Table 4.1); however, in some of these conditions, they do not normally disappear even when the primary cause is removed. In this chapter, which represents a sort of compendium as well as a continuation of the previous one, I will illustrate the morphological features of substances which, unlike water, glycogen, and lipids (represented by achromatic material), are composed of stained and/or granular material that becomes recognizable with the application of standard stains. There are also extracytoplasmic accumulations (Table 4.2) with specific shapes and colors, whose diagnostic identification is of fundamental importance for effective evaluation of cytological samples. Some materials, such as bile, are more easily recognized by cytological (rather than histological) investigation, and they do not even require the use of special stains. In light of the above, I will continue to consider the cytological investigation as preparatory to and dependent on the histopathological diagnostic process. In this chapter, the features of these accumulations are described because they are essential for several diagnoses.

4.1   Pathological Intracytoplasmic Accumulation

4.1.1   Lipofuscin

Cytomorphology: cytoplasmic, bluish to greenish pigment, dispersed in the cytoplasm in variable amounts, sometimes very abundant (Figure 4.1); may be observed in clumps (Figure 4.2).

Canine and Feline Liver Cytology, First Edition. Carlo Masserdotti.
© 2024 John Wiley & Sons, Inc. Published 2024 by John Wiley & Sons, Inc.

Table 4.1 Identification of intracytoplasmic accumulation.

	Lipofuscin	Copper	Iron and hemosiderin	Protein droplets	Eosinophilic granules	Storage diseases
Color	Blue	Teal colored, refractile	From golden-brown to bluish-black	Slightly blue	Pink to red	Achromatic globules
Shape and dimension	Granular small	Granular small	Small to large clumps	Globular large	Granular small	Round, small to medium sized
Location	Hepatocytes	Hepatocytes	Hepatocytes and macrophages	Hepatocytes	Hepatocytes	Hepatocytes
Interpretation	Oxidative stress, aging	Possible copper toxicosis	Hemophagocytosis	ER stress	Many primary diseases	Inherited, sometimes acquired metabolic enzyme deficiencies

Table 4.2 Identification of extracytoplasmic accumulation.

	Bile	Amyloid
Color	Green-blue to blue-black	Pink to orange
Shape	Elongated casts	Irregular tufts
Location	Among hepatocytes	Around hepatocytes sheet
Interpretation	Cholestasis	Amyloidosis

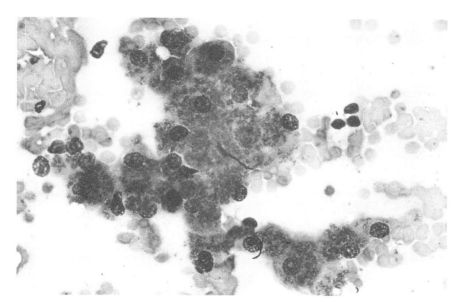

Figure 4.1 Normal liver, FNCS, dog. A large amount of bluish-green pigment into the cytoplasm of otherwise normal hepatocytes (MGG, 100×).

This is by far the most common accumulation found in the hepatocyte cytoplasm. It can be useful for hepatocyte identification if the hepatic parenchyma is widely replaced by metastatic neoplastic cells or whenever it is difficult to recognize hepatocytes (for example, when the hepatocytes are embedded in bloody material). Lipofuscin may look different, more or less basophilic depending on the selected stain method (Figure 4.3). Lipofuscin may be present in normal and injured hepatocytes, where the pigment is dispersed into the cytoplasm together with achromatic material (water or glycogen – Figure 4.4) or among the lipid globules (Figure 4.5); lipofuscin may also accumulate in hepatocytes when other unrelated pathological conditions occur, such as extracytoplasmic cholestasis

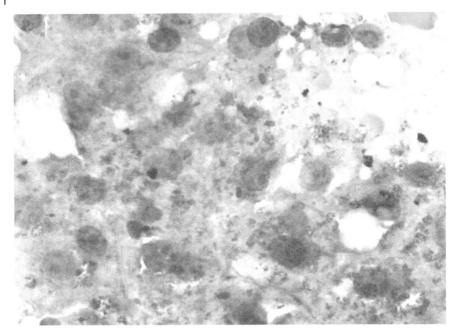

Figure 4.2 Normal liver, FNCS, dog. Lipofuscin aggregates, inside the cytoplasm of some cells, in small clumps (Hemacolor®, 100×).

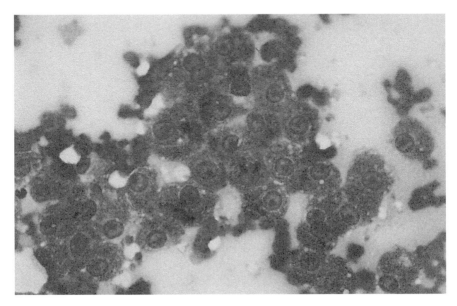

Figure 4.3 Normal liver, FNCS, dog. Notice that lipofuscin looks different with Romanowsky stains than with MGG (Diff-Quik®, 100×).

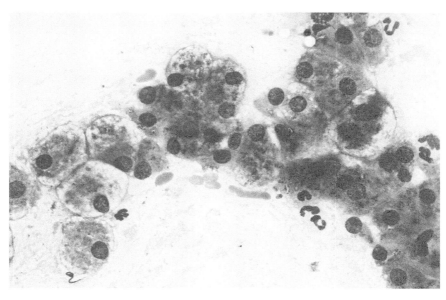

Figure 4.4 Liver, reversible hepatic injury, FNCS, dog. Lipofuscin may be observed inside the cytoplasm of cells affected by reversible injury, as water or glycogen accumulation (MGG, 100×).

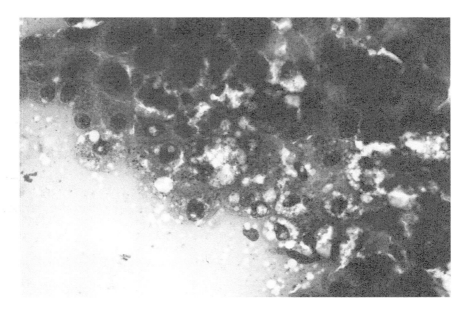

Figure 4.5 Liver, reversible hepatic injury, FNCS, cat. Lipofuscin may be observed inside the cytoplasm of hepatocytes filled with fat globules (MGG, 100×).

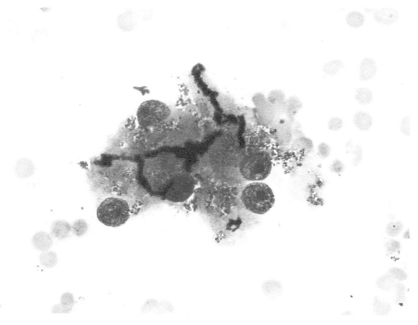

Figure 4.6 Liver, cholestasis, dog. A small group of hepatocytes, with cytoplasm filled with lipofuscin; notice the casts of biliary material among the cells' borders and the difference in colors (MGG, 100×).

(Figure 4.6). The amount of lipofuscin pigment may depend on the nature of the injury; for example, oxidant injury induced by copper deposition will produce accumulation of a large amount of pigment.

In ultrastructural examinations, lipofuscin is represented by a pigment that accumulates inside the lysosomes. This pigment results from oxidation processes mediated by the activity of lysosomal hydrolases on phospholipids, which presumably come from membranous residues of cytoplasmic organelles, concentrated in the form of undigested residual body [1]. This phenomenon is the consequence of very limited (sometimes even negligible) and nonspecific degenerative processes, such as increased cell turnover. Although the presence of lipofuscin is considered to be mostly unrelated to pathological implications, in samples from elderly subjects it can accumulate in very large amounts [2]. Lipofuscin is nearly always present in hepatocytes of cats after a few years of age. In light of the above, lipofuscin has also been called the "aging pigment" or the "wear and tear pigment" as it tends to accumulate later in life and prematurely with chronic liver injury as a consequence of increased cell turnover [3]. Lipofuscin, as phospholipid debris, may also accumulate in lysosomes if their activity is reduced by alkalinization of the lysosomal interior [3] or if lysosomal hydrolase is genetically defective [4]. Accumulations of lipofuscin in humans, dogs, and mice can develop as a consequence of exposure to amiodarone, an antiarrhythmic drug that causes alterations in the pH for hydrolase functionality [5].

Due to its chromatic similarity, in the past lipofuscin was mistakenly believed to be a cytoplasmic accumulation of bile [6]. However, lipofuscin is unrelated to intracytoplasmic biliary stasis. Furthermore, as previously stated, it is virtually impossible to evaluate bile accumulation in cytoplasm by cytological investigation. The enlightening results of research conducted by Scott and Buriko [7], carried out with special stains and electron microscopy, have excluded a biliary derivation. This study relegates lipofuscin to a virtually harmless role with no diagnostic implications, except enhanced oxidative damage. It is important to recall that, depending on the quality of standard stains, lipofuscin may appear as bluish to greenish pigment [8] and may accumulate in the cytoplasm, sometimes in large clumped basophilic granules; in these cases, care must be taken to exclude cholestasis, which is generally represented by basophilic casts among hepatocytes and never by cytoplasmic accumulation.

The presence of lipofuscin can also occur in neoplastic hepatocytes. It has been reported in small amounts in cells of a well-differentiated hepatocellular carcinoma [9].

4.1.2 Copper

Cytomorphology: presence of indistinct, blurred, teal-colored, slightly refractile granules, sometimes with a crystal-like appearance. Granules can accumulate in small to abundant amounts in the cytoplasm (Figures 4.7 and 4.8); most often hepatocytes are otherwise normal. Occasionally, hepatocytes exhibit variable degree of dilation because of accumulated indistinct achromatic material or lipid globules; association with inflammatory cells and with fibrosis features is an occasional finding (Figure 4.9).

Recognition of the morphological features of copper accumulation is quite difficult with standard stain methods but may be quite evident with rhodanine stain (Figure 4.10). The affected hepatocyte cytoplasm may also contain small amounts of associated material of achromatic, dispersed or globular appearance [10]; associated accumulation of lipofuscin is also possible.

Injury from copper accumulation, which in the English literature is defined as "copper toxicosis," is a pathological process that may occur in a variety of dog breeds and occasionally cats. It is suspected that dietary copper is a major source of excess hepatic copper. There are genetic metabolic defects affecting some dog breeds. The best known mutation occurs in the Bedlington terrier, in which a genetic mutation in the COMM-D1 gene produces a defective protein, involved in cytoplasmic copper transport into bile with the consequent accumulation of intracytoplasmic copper [11]. Labrador retrievers may experience a syndrome of

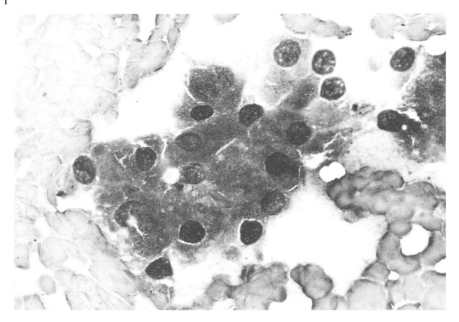

Figure 4.7 Liver, copper toxicosis, FNCS, dog. Blurred, teal-colored, slightly refractile granules of copper accumulated in the cytoplasm (MGG, 100×).

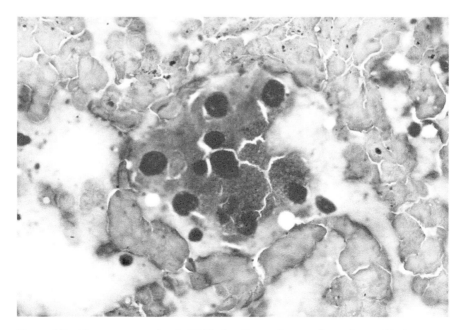

Figure 4.8 Liver, copper toxicosis, FNCS, dog. Copper is sometimes clumped in large teal-colored granules (MGG, 100×).

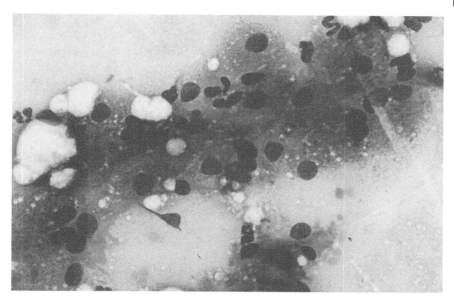

Figure 4.9   Liver, copper toxicosis, FNCS, dog. Copper-filled hepatocytes arranged around strands of spindle cells (MGG, 100×).

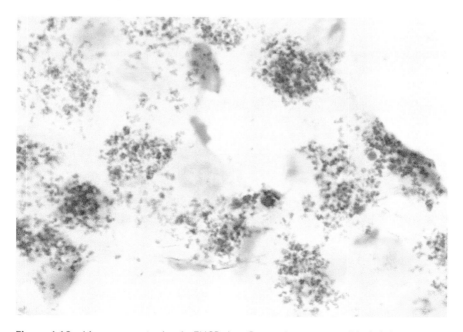

Figure 4.10   Liver, copper toxicosis, FNCS, dog. Copper is represented by bright orange granules with special stain (rhodanine, 100×).

hepatic copper excess that is associated with mutations in the ATP7a and ATP7b genes [12]. Other breeds such as the West Highland white terrier, Skye terrier, Dobermann pinscher, and Dalmatian have an increased risk of copper excess but the genetics are not well characterized [13]. Mixed-breed dogs and occasionally cats can develop hepatic copper excess [14]. Excess copper causes hepatocyte oxidative damage, which can lead to reversible nonspecific damage; its persistence over time represents approximately one-third of the causes of chronic hepatitis, a disease with irreversible and progressive evolution.

The diagnosis for copper toxicosis is based on the overall amount of hepatic copper. In the initial stages, accumulation normally involves the centrilobular and subsequently midzonal segments, although all hepatocytes can be affected. Ultimately, liver copper values, investigated with inductively coupled plasma atomic emission spectroscopy (ICP-AES), are the most informative [15, 16]. By this method, a median hepatic concentration of 1274 µg/g (563.0–1773.0) in predisposed breeds and 542.2 µg/g (270.3–862.3) in nonpredisposed breeds seems to be correlated with hepatitis [16].

Copper is eliminated via the bile and a small amount of copper may be seen secondary to cholestasis and in cases of chronic hepatitis [8, 17]. According to other data, copper accumulation does not seem to be enhanced by cholestasis in dogs [18]. In this case, it remains to be established whether copper accumulation is primary or secondary to chronic inflammation, fibrosis or cholestasis [19]. Cytology can estimate the proportion of affected hepatocytes, but it is clear that only histological investigation with precise indications about the localization of copper accumulation is useful to identify the extent of copper retention in hepatocytes. Consequently, cytological examination has no diagnostic application other than the identification of suspicious material in the cytoplasm, represented by irregular water-green granules in variable quantities.

Routine cytological staining may be ineffective in recognizing cytoplasmic copper so special stains such as rhodanine, widely accepted as more reliable and simple, or rubeanic acid must be applied [8, 20]. Cytoplasmic copper–protein complexes stain blue-green to green-black with rubeanic acid and bright orange-red with rhodanine. This allows confirmation of the presence of cytoplasmic copper, as well as an opportunity to carry out a semiquantitative evaluation [21]. Orcein [22] and Timm's silver sulfide stain [23] have also been used to identify copper, although no data on cytological samples have been published.

4.1.3 Iron and Hemosiderin

Cytomorphology: presence of coarse, dense, sometimes clumped cytoplasmic granules, which accumulate mainly in the cytoplasm of activated Kupffer cells; the color ranges from golden-brown to bluish-black (Figures 4.11–4.14); possible to observe accumulation of similar material in the cytoplasm of hepatocytes (Figure 4.15).

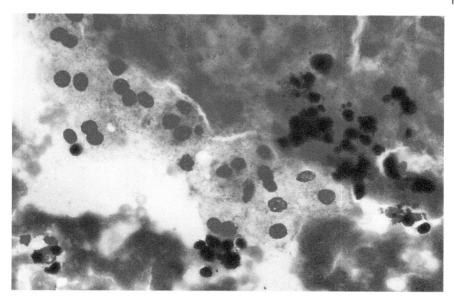

Figure 4.11 Liver, mild anemia of chronic disease, FNCS, dog. Kupffer cells with indistinct cytoplasm filled with golden-brown material, in large clumps, surround and infiltrate an aggregate of normal hepatocytes (MGG, 100×).

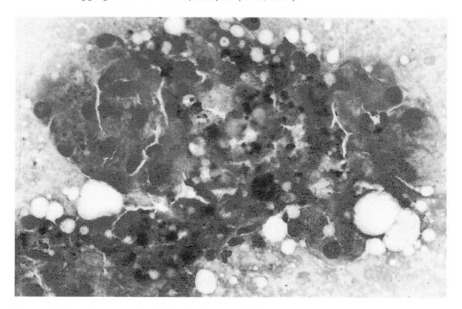

Figure 4.12 Liver, anemia of chronic disease, FNCS, dog. A group of Kupffer cells that show erythrophagocytosis and phagocytosis of bluish granular material embedded in a hepatocyte aggregate (MGG, 100×).

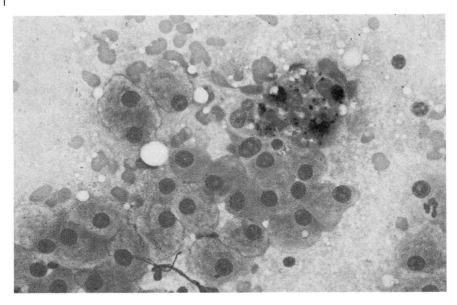

Figure 4.13 Liver, anemia of chronic disease, FNCS, dog. A group of Kupffer cells with indistinct cytoplasm and a high amount of brown to bluish clumped material, aggregated on top of slightly dilated hepatocytes (MGG, 100×).

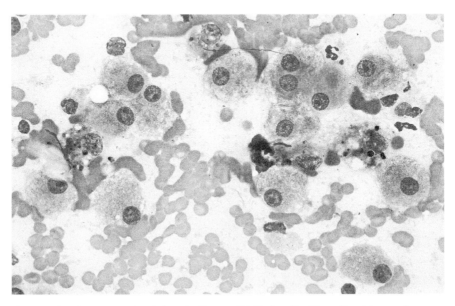

Figure 4.14 Liver, anemia of chronic disease, FNCS, dog. Kupffer cells with cytoplasm filled with brown (central) to bluish (on the sides) material, scattered among slightly dilated hepatocytes (MGG, 100×).

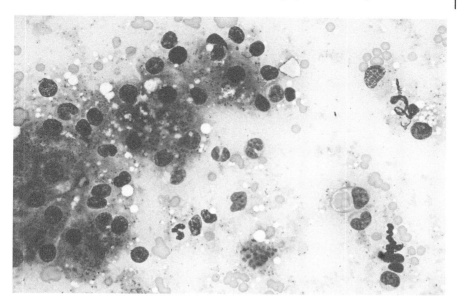

Figure 4.15   Liver, centrilobular congestion, FNCS, dog. The hepatocytes on the top of the aggregate are filled with a moderate amount of brownish granular material; compare this material with lipofuscin in the cytoplasm of hepatocytes at the bottom. On the right side, a Kupffer cell shows erythrophagocytosis (MGG, 100×).

This cytoplasmatic material is produced by the Kupffer cells as they digest the hemoglobin contained in the red blood cells, which are phagocytized when they exit the vascular lumina as a consequence of senescence, immune-mediated destruction, red blood cell infections, congestive or hemorrhagic conditions (Figures 4.16 and 4.17); Prussian blue stain helps in identification of iron pigment, which looks bright blue (Figure 4.18). Centrilobular and sinusoidal congestion, induced for example by alteration of venous outflow, as in the case of right-sided heart failure or chronic cardiomyopathies [24] or as a consequence of mechanical extrahepatic obstructions or subobstructions (for example, neoplasms) [25], may also be followed by stasis of erythrocytes, which may be removed and destroyed by Kupffer cells.

Common causes of erythrophagocytosis or hemosiderosis includes anemia of chronic diseases or chronic hepatitis [2]. Similar to the spleen, the liver is a hemocatheretic organ, so erythrosiderophagocytosis events may also occur as a consequence of immune-mediated hemolytic events (the most frequent causes of erythrocyte destruction), which in turn are induced by primary causes [26]. The causes of erythrocyte destruction also include hemolytic anemia with secondary hemochromatosis, described in the dog [27], where an accumulation of hemosiderin granules occurs in the cytoplasm of Kupffer cells and hepatocytes. Erythrocatheresis performed by macrophages can sometimes be associated with

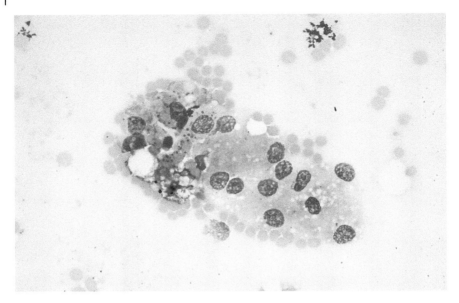

Figure 4.16   Liver, centrilobular congestion, FNCS, dog. A group of Kupffer cells with enlarged cytoplasm, filled with brownish granular material and red blood cells (MGG, 100×).

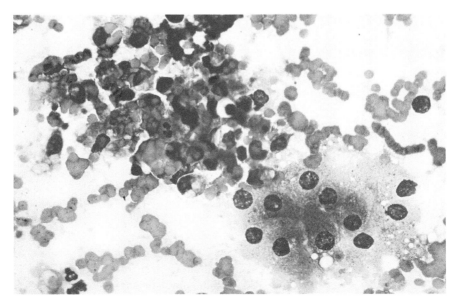

Figure 4.17   Liver, microhemorrhagia and venous congestion, FNCS, dog. A large aggregate of Kupffer cells that show erythrophagocytosis (MGG, 100×).

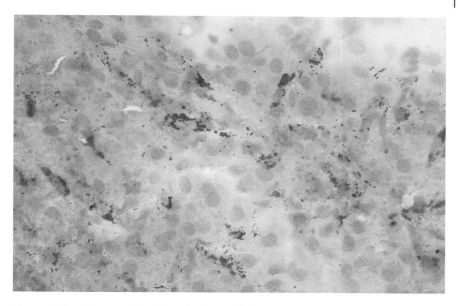

Figure 4.18   Liver, anemia of chronic disease, FNCS, dog. Iron pigment looks blue when stained with special stain (Prussian blue, 100×).

chronic inflammatory conditions of the liver parenchyma, probably as a consequence of focal necrosis, parenchymal microhemorrhage, and macrophage removal. Destruction of red cells leading to chronic anemia and administration of iron-based compounds or repeated transfusions are other possible causes [28].

A very rare disease, known as erythropoietic protoporphyria, is caused by an excess of protoporphyrin, normally involved in heme synthesis. Protoporphyrin accepts Fe^{++} ions from the enzyme ferrochelatase in the heme biosynthesis pathway, but it accumulates as a consequence of partial deficiency of ferrochelatase activity. Protoporphyrin is released in the plasma and taken up by the liver and vascular endothelium. Protoporphyrin is recognizable as dark brown pigment in canaliculi and interlobular bile ducts and, in severe cases, also in Kupffer cells; it has a characteristic Maltese cross form when viewed under polarized light. Deposition of pigment may result in chronic hepatitis and cirrhosis.

This condition can be acquired and may result from the use of drugs such as griseofulvin or a drug used in the treatment of arthritis (3-[2-(2, 4, 6 trimethylphenyl)-thiothyl]methylsydnone – TTMS) [2]; however, an association with antipsychotic drugs has also been indicated, though only at experimental level [29]. A transient form of protoporphyria was observed in a group of 17 dogs (German shepherds, belonging to the same breeder), probably due to exposure to unknown substances with porphyrinogenic and inhibitory action of the iron chelatase enzyme [30].

Finally, in addition to the exogenous causes described, a form of congenital protoporphyria has been described [31].

4.1.4 Protein Droplets

Cytomorphology: weakly basophilic hyaline globules, with an irregularly rounded or polygonal profile and cytoplasmic accumulation, with a tendency to deform the nucleus and displace other globular achromatic material (Figure 4.19).

Described as a consequence of shock events, ischemia or associated with hepatocellular damage, this is a rare condition. The cause is unclear but one theory is that it is caused by accumulation of protein plasma-derived material; another explanation is that alterations in the function of the endoplasmic reticulum (ER) can result in the accumulation of unfolded or misfolded proteins, a cellular condition referred to as ER stress [32]. I have personally observed it in a case of hepatocarcinoma [33].

4.1.5 Cytoplasmic Granular Eosinophilic Material

Cytomorphology: small granular eosinophilic globules of variable size (Figure 4.20), sometimes coalescing in aggregates with an irregular profile (Figures 4.21–4.23).

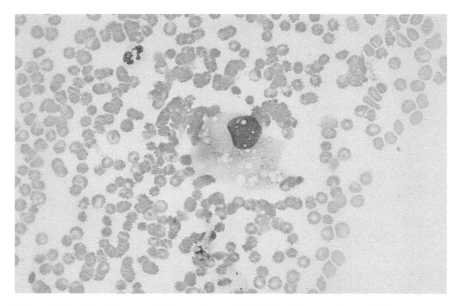

Figure 4.19 Liver, hepatocellular carcinoma, FNCS, dog. The cytoplasm of this hepatocyte is filled with large, slight blue globules with distinct borders and roundish shape, that displace the nuclear outline (MGG, 100×).

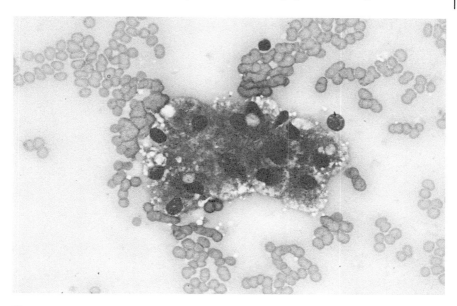

Figure 4.20   Liver, aspecific hepatitis, FNCS, dog. The cytoplasm of this hepatocytes is filled with lipid globules and small eosinophilic granules (MGG, 100×).

Figure 4.21   Liver, aspecific hepatitis, FNCS, dog. Small eosinophilic granules inside the cytoplasm of some hepatocytes that coalesce in larger globules (MGG, 100×).

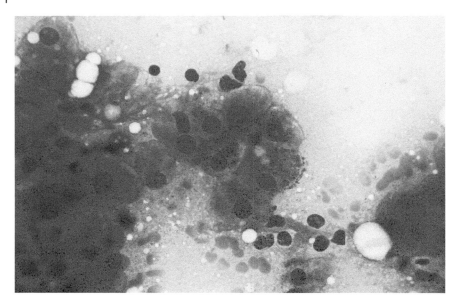

Figure 4.22 Liver, aspecific hepatitis, FNCS, dog. In rare cases, it is possible to observe eosinophilic granules inside the cytoplasm of hepatocytes surrounded by inflammatory cells (MGG, 100×).

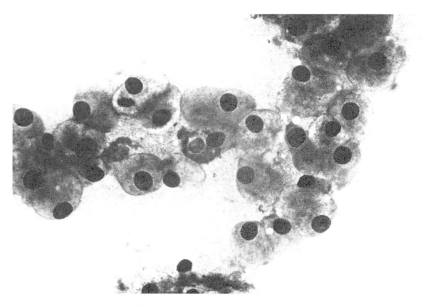

Figure 4.23 Liver, aspecific hepatitis, FNCS, dog. Granules may condense in large, irregularly shaped cytoplasmic aggregates (MGG, 100×).

In human medicine, some distinct conditions are known; the eosinophilic granules that accumulate in the cytoplasm may be represented by macroglobules (mainly Mallory–Denk bodies) and microglobules (the accumulation of alpha-1-antitrypsin, alpha-1-fetoprotein, haptoglobin or alpha-macroglobulin), sometimes also observed in the dog with chronic liver diseases. Among macroglobules, Mallory–Denk bodies are irregular, dense cytoplasmic inclusions with a cytokeratin component, often in the form of strands or garlands that sometimes form a ring around the nucleus; electron microscopy reveals that Mallory–Denk bodies are protein aggregates bundled with intermediate filaments; in humans the presence of Mallory–Denk bodies has been associated with many conditions, including degenerative changes, chronic cholestasis, drug-induced damage, preneoplastic conditions, and benign and malignant hepatocellular neoplasms [34]. Although it remains unclear whether Mallory–Denk bodies serve a bystander, protective or injury-promoting function, they have an important role as histological and potential progression markers in several liver diseases in humans. Although they have never been described previously in veterinary cytology, personal observation suggests that eosinophilic bodies with morphological features identical to Mallory–Denk bodies were observed in liver of the dog.

Among the microglobules, deficiency of alpha-1-antitrypsin (AAT) has long been known to cause liver cirrhosis in humans. AAT, a serine proteinase inhibitor, blocks the enzymatic activity of many proteases [35]; the defect is one in which AAT, which is normally produced in the liver, cannot be secreted into the blood and therefore accumulates within hepatocytes, causing chronic damage [36]. Whether the same mechamism occurs in dog is uncertain, although AAT has been previously described [37].

In dogs and cats, cytological identification of eosinophilic globules is easy. There are no specific pathological conditions that can explain the accumulation of these extremely rare materials, although chronic inflammatory conditions should be considered. The presence of small eosinophilic globules does not exclude hepatic neoplasia, since they have been identified in small amounts in the cytoplasm of hepatocytes of well-differentiated hepatocellular carcinoma [9].

Other cytoplasmic inclusions may be the result of phagocytosis of apoptotic bodies by hepatocytes [38], although no cytological description is available in the literature.

4.1.6 Hepatic Lysosomal Storage Disorders

This group of very rare diseases may be associated with inherited or sometimes acquired metabolic enzymes deficiencies. Lysosomal storage refers to a cellular alteration in which an increased amount of material that is normally degraded accumulates within the lysosomes of cells, often resulting in cell death. The disease is thought to result from mutations causing a reduction in lysosomal enzyme synthesis. The most common finding is the presence of clear true vacuoles sometimes containing hyaline, granular or pigmented granules in hepatocytes and/or Kupffer cells; this change is due to the accumulation of fucose, ganglio-sides, glycosil ceramines, mucopolysaccharides [39], sphingomyelin, unesteri-fied cholesterol, and other factors. No descriptions of cytological features have been published but the suspicion should occur whenever evidence of unex-plained globules in the cytoplasm of hepatocytes is observed; this disease may associate with similar changes in other cells such as brain cells or circulating blood cells.

4.2 Pathological Extracytoplasmic Accumulation

4.2.1 Bile

Cytomorphology: linear or branched casts that follow the profile of the hepato-cytes' cytoplasmic membranes, with a dark green-blue to blue-black color (Figure 4.24); frequent association with reversible nonspecific hepatocellular damage, represented by accumulation of lipofuscin (Figure 4.25), water, glycogen or lipids (Figure 4.26); sometimes association with macrophages that phagocytize bile released from canaliculi (Figure 4.27). There may also be a variable amount of inflammatory cells, generally related to primary causes (Figure 4.28).

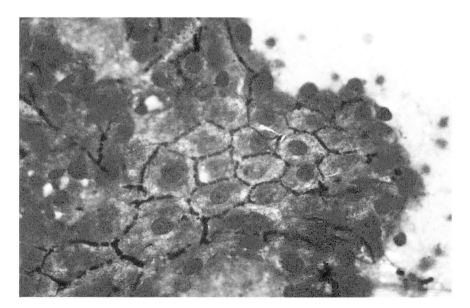

Figure 4.24 Liver, cholestasis, FNCS, dog. Branched casts of bluish-greenish biliary material among the cytoplasmic borders of hepatocytes (MGG, 100×).

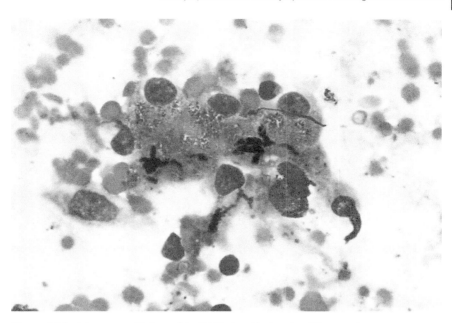

Figure 4.25 Liver, aspecific hepatitis, FNCS, dog. Notice the difference between lipofuscin, represented by bluish granular material inside the cytoplasm, and bile, represented by linear casts outside the cytoplasm (MGG, 100×).

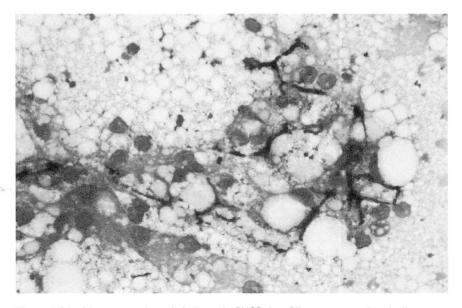

Figure 4.26 Liver, steatosis and cholestasis, FNCS, dog. Bile can accumulate in linear casts among hepatocytes enlarged by lipid globules (MGG, 100×).

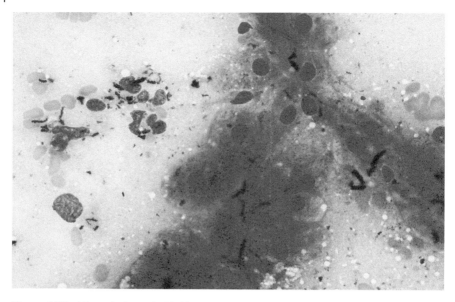

Figure 4.27 Liver, cholestasis, FNCS, dog. An aggregate of hepatocytes crossed by linear casts of bile; notice the macrophages on the left side, with cytoplasm filled with the same material (MGG, 100×).

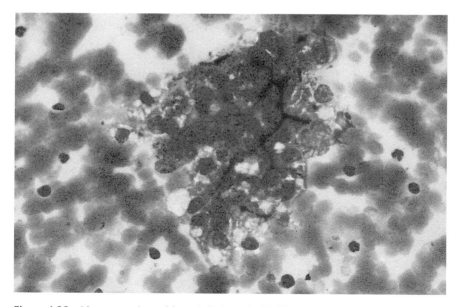

Figure 4.28 Liver, acute hepatitis and cholestasis, FNCS, dog. Hepatocytes surrounded by inflammatory cells, mostly represented by well-preserved neutrophils and crossed by branched casts of bile (MGG, 100×).

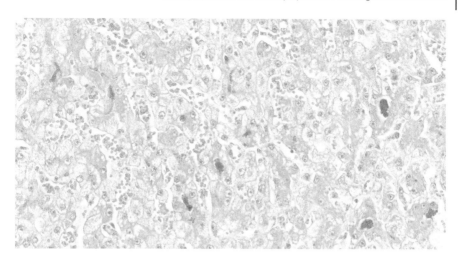

Figure 4.29   Liver, cholestasis, FNCS, dog. Bile is difficult to recognize in histological section, mostly when in low amounts or focal and represented by yellow-greenish casts (HE, 40×).

Identifying extracytoplasmic cholestasis histologically featuring linear or branched casts of pale green biliary material between hepatocytes can be difficult (Figure 4.29). In contrast, detection of extracytoplasmic accumulation of bile is quite a satisfactory moment in the evaluation of a cytological preparation of the liver, as it provides clear, easy, and incontrovertible (especially when widespread and abundant) information relating to alterations in the outflow of the bile itself. The bilirubin and bile acids, metabolized in the hepatocellular cytoplasm, are transferred by transmembrane carrier proteins in the biliary canaliculi. The latter, very thin intercytoplasmic linear cavities found between two adjacent plates of hepatocytes can be histologically assessed only when they dilate during cholestasis. Through these cavities, the bile flows against the blood flow, from the centrilobular segments to the portal ones, reaching the short segments called the canals of Hering and finally the increasingly larger interlobular bile ducts in the portal tracts, the large extrahepatic ducts, the gallbladder, the common bile duct and the intestinal outlet, represented by the duodenal papilla. Any intra- or extrahepatic obstructive condition to the normal outflow of bile can cause cholestasis – from hepatocytic swelling (such as lipidosis) to obstruction of the biliary tract. Any mechanical extrahepatic obstruction, especially masses, lymph node enlargements, gallstones, parasites, primary or secondary biliary diseases or occlusion of duodenal papilla, must be investigated by radiographic or ultrasonographic examination.

It should be noted that the cause of the obstruction may be localized in selected or focal areas of the biliary tract or the hepatic parenchyma, such as a localized neoplasm; in these cases (involving only specific areas of the liver), the cytological survey of cholestasis is successful only if the sampling is carried out from the parenchymal segments involved.

Generalized cholestasis involving the entire parenchyma is often (and easily) observed:

- if the obstructive damage is localized in the large terminal ducts, as in the case of enlargement of the hilar lymph nodes, or in the presence of hepatic or extra-hepatic neoplastic masses or occlusion of the lumen of major bile ducts
- in case of stones or in the course of cystic mucinous hyperplasia of the gallbladder, if mucus occludes the common bile duct
- in case of occlusion of the duodenal papilla, typically in the course of severe inflammation of the intestinal mucosa, neoplasia or the presence of foreign bodies.

It should also be noted that a mechanical occlusion may not be visible and that cholestatic events can occur due to marked swelling of the hepatocytes, for example following severe nonspecific and reversible damage [40].

Other causes of cholestasis could include a form of fulminant hepatitis, forms of subacute or chronic hepatitis with cirrhosis or induced by hemolytic anemia that both increases the load for bilirubin synthesis and impairs the ability of hepatocytes to function due to hypoxia and centrilobular necrosis [41]. In these cases, the most likely cause of cholestasis is linked to perturbation induced by the pathological process that destroys the normal microarchitecture of the canalicular outflow system. Similarly, many forms of hepatitis with cholestasis are induced by viral, bacterial or parasitic etiological agents – further discussed in the following chapters.

The cytological evidence of cholestasis is therefore nonspecific and detection should activate all clinical investigations. Hematological data concerning severe anemia and liver-specific enzymes, which are indicative of liver damage or insufficiency, as well as imaging investigations, can all be useful to identify the site and causes of the disrupted bile flow.

4.2.2 Amyloid

Cytomorphology: presence of eosinophilic, dense fibrillar material in tufts and bundles of varying thickness, which accumulate between the aggregates of hepatocytes (Figure 4.30). This material may disrupt the epithelial sheets and accumulate on the background of the smear; possible association with chronic mild, mostly histiocytic inflammation (Figure 4.31). Phagocytosis of amyloid from macrophages may be observed (Figure 4.32); hepatocytes look generally normal (Figure 4.33).

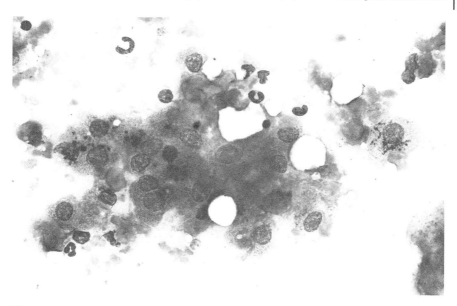

Figure 4.30   Liver, amyloidosis, FNCS, cat. Tufts of dense, eosinophilic amyloid accumulate among the hepatocytes (MGG, 100×).

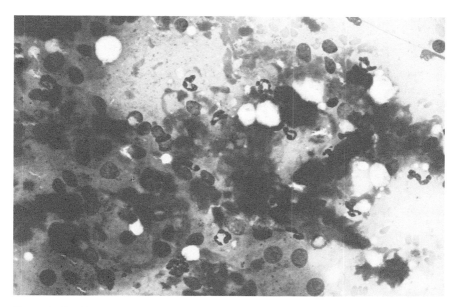

Figure 4.31   Liver, amyloidosis, FNCS, cat. A large amount of amyloid, represented by aggregates of extracytoplasmic eosinophilic material that surround a cluster of hepatocytes, together with inflammatory cells (MGG, 100×).

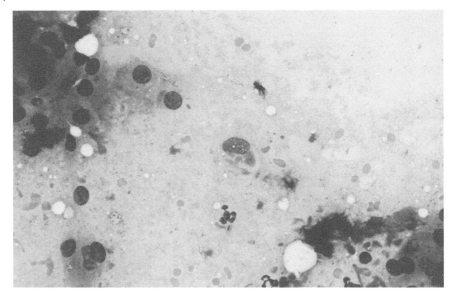

Figure 4.32 Liver, amyloidosis, FNCS, cat. A single Kupffer cell, with cytoplasm filled with eosinophilic, dense amyloid (MGG, 100×).

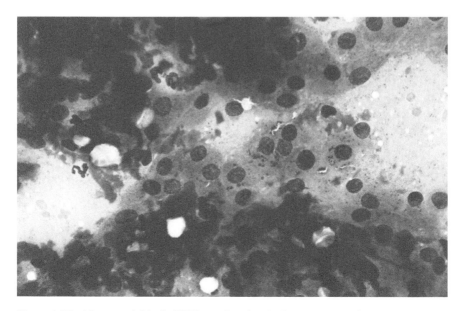

Figure 4.33 Liver, amyloidosis, FNCS, cat. Despite the large amount of amyloid that accumulates in large tufts, hepatocytes look normal or are filled with a small amount of lipofuscin (MGG, 100×).

Often, in books or specialized reviews, it is stated that recognition of amyloid is possible only with the use of special stains, together with observation with polarized light. Personally, I find these investigations superfluous in the context of a practical diagnosis, as the morphological features of this material (previously described) and its abundant quantities make the recognition of this process fairly easy. Inexperienced cytologists may have to learn to distinguish amyloid from proteinaceous debris, such as amorphous eosinophilic or basophilic material (Figure 4.34) and especially platelet aggregates (Figure 4.35), which can be identified on the base of their corpuscular features. Amyloid may be difficult to recognize, without special stains, in histological sections (Figure 4.36).

It is also advisable to distinguish amyloid from hepatic fibrosis, which tends to have peculiar morphological features (Figure 4.37), as described in Chapter 8. Indeed, spindle cells, if embedded in bundles of fibrillary stroma, may resemble the focal deposition of amyloid. Another common artifact to be distinguished from amyloid is the artifactual distribution among the hepatic cells of the gel used for ultrasonographic examination (Figure 4.38).

Amyloid, a protein formed by peptides folded into beta-pleated sheets, has a structure that features dense fibrils. Several protein precursors are known, but the liver-localized amyloid deposits generally include amyloid resulting from light chain proteins (AL amyloid) or from proteins synthesized directly from the

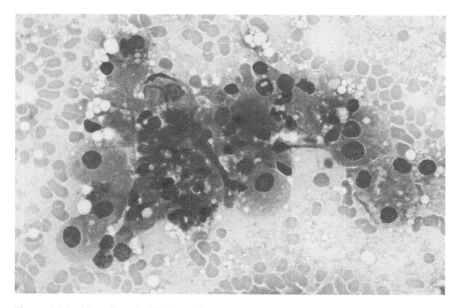

Figure 4.34 Liver, fibrosis, FNCS, cat. Dense eosinophilic material, focally fibrillar, probably of stromal origin, surrounding some inflammatory cells and accumulated among hepatocytes (MGG, 100×).

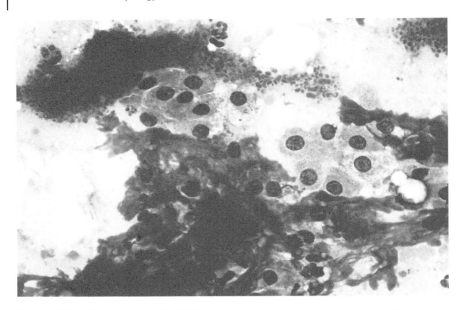

Figure 4.35 Liver, amyloidosis, FNCS, dog. Compare the amyloid represented by large, fibrillar and branched tufts in the center of the image and the large aggregate of platelets on the top (MGG, 100×).

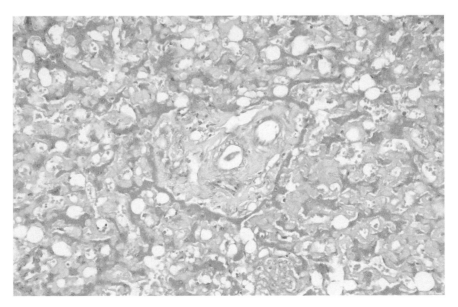

Figure 4.36 Liver, amyloidosis, FNCS, cat. In histological section amyloid looks like bundles of dense, eosinophilic, homogeneous material, but its recognition is difficult without special stains (HE, 40×).

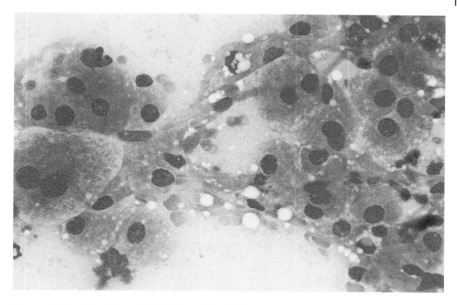

Figure 4.37 Liver, fibrosis, FNCS, dog. Fibrosis is represented by strands of fibrillary material, frequently crossed by spindle nucleated cells (MGG, 100×).

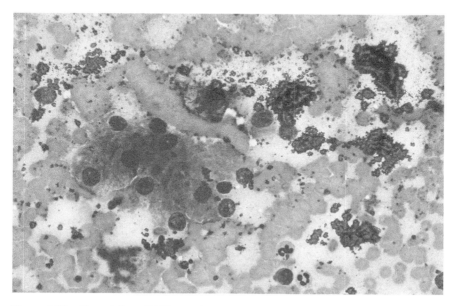

Figure 4.38 Normal liver, FNCS, dog. Gel used for ultrasonographic examination may pollute the smear and looks like amyloid; notice the granular, pink, crystalline material irregularly scattered on the background (MGG, 100×).

hepatocyte (AA amyloid). AA amyloid arises from an acute-phase protein which, when produced in pathological amounts as a consequence of chronic inflammatory processes, tends to accumulate in folded sheets, mainly in the interstitial area of the space of Disse but also in the vascular wall, the interstitium or glomeruli of the renal parenchyma and sometimes in the splenic parenchyma (intra- or perivascular). The association with chronic extrahepatic inflammatory diseases – to be assessed by detailed clinical and anamnestic research and possibly, in the cat, by comparison with the dosage level of serum amyloid (SAA) – should always be regarded as the most likely cause of amyloidosis, especially when the inflammatory condition is difficult to prove [42].

Amyloid accumulation can also occur due to hereditary predisposition which, in the cat, can be found mostly in the Abyssinian and Siamese breeds and, in dogs, in the shar pei or chow-chow. However, any breed can be affected in the presence of chronic inflammation disease. In cats, amyloidosis is not breed limited and it is also described in the domestic short hair and Devon rex [43, 44]. In some rare conditions, amyloid is deposited by neoplastic plasma cells as a consequence of protein overproduction, as reported in a cat with extramedullary plasmacytoma [45].

4.3 Key Points

- Lipofuscin, although considered to be a very slight cytoplasmic change, is normally present inside the cytoplasm of hepatocyte, irrespective of the amount present.
- Copper toxicosis, when suspected by the cytological evidence of copper accumulation in the cytoplasm of hepatocytes, must be always confirmed by histological and histochemical methods.
- Iron and hemosiderin accumulation are frequent findings; when present, first consider increased hemocatheretic activity of the liver, as a consequence of red blood cell turnover.
- Bile cast accumulation among hepatocytes is a reliable method for assessing cholestasis; when present, first consider causes of bile flow obstruction.
- Cytological features are pathognomonic for amyloidosis; when present, there is no need for further investigation.

References

1 Goldfischer, S. and Bernstein, J. (1969). Lipofuscin (aging) pigment granules of the newborn human liver. *J. Cell Biol.* 42 (1): 253–261.
2 Van Winkle, T., Ullen, J.M., van den Ingh, T.S.G.A.M. et al. (2006). Morphological classification of parenchymal disorders of the canine and feline liver – hepatic

abscess and granulomas, hepatic metabolic storage disorders and miscellaneous conditions. In: *Standard for Clinical and Histological Diagnosis of Canine and Feline Liver Disease* (ed. WSAVA Liver Standardization Group), 106–109. St Louis, MO: Saunders.

3 Hayes, A.M. (2004). Pathophysiology of the liver. In: *Veterinary Pathophysiology* (ed. R. Dunlop and C. Malbert), 382. Ames, IA: Blackwell Publishing.

4 Warren, C.D. and Alroy, J. (2000). Morphological, biochemical and molecular biology approaches for the diagnosis of lysosomal storage diseases. *J. Vet. Diagn. Invest.* 12 (6): 483–496.

5 Schneider, P. (1992). Drug-induced lysosomal disorders in laboratory animals. New substances acting on lysosomes. *Arch. Toxicol.* 62: 23–33.

6 Perman, V., Alasker, R.D., and Riis, R.C. (1979). *Cytology of the Dog and Cat*, 152–153. South Bend, IN: American Animal Hospital Association.

7 Scott, M. and Buriko, K. (2005). Characterization of the pigmented cytoplasmic granules common in canine hepatocytes. *Vet. Clin. Pathol.* 34 (suppl): 281–282.

8 Arndt, T.P. and Shelly, S.M. (2014). The liver. In: *Diagnostic Cytology of the Dog and Cat*, 4e (ed. A.C. Valenciano and R.L. Cowell), 354–371. St Louis, MO: Elsevier Mosby.

9 Masserdotti, C. and Drigo, M. (2012). Retrospective study of cytologic features of well-differentiated hepatocellular carcinoma in dogs. *Vet. Clin. Pathol.* 41 (3): 382–390.

10 Meyer, D.K. (2016). The liver. In: *Canine and Feline Cytology – A Color Atlas and Interpretation Guide*, 3e (ed. R.E. Raskin and D.J. Meyer), 259–283. St Louis, MO: Elsevier.

11 Forman, O.P., Boursnell, M.E.G., Dunmore, B.J. et al. (2005). Characterization of the COMMD1 (MURR1) mutation causing copper toxicosis in Bedlington terriers. *Anim. Genet.* 36 (6): 497–501.

12 Wu, X., den Boer, E.R., Vos-Loohuis, M. et al. (2020). Investigation of genetic modifiers of copper toxicosis in Labrador retrievers. *Life* 10 (11): 266.

13 Rodrigues, A., Leal, R.O., Girod, M. et al. (2020). Canine copper-associated hepatitis: a retrospective study of 17 clinical cases. *Open Vet. J.* 10 (2): 128–134.

14 Whittemore, J.C., Newkirk, K.M., Reel, D.M., and Reed, A. (2012). Hepatic copper and iron accumulation and histologic findings in 104 feline liver biopsies. *J. Vet. Diagn. Invest.* 24 (4): 656–661.

15 Smedley, R., Mullaney, R., and Rumbeiha, W. (2009). Copper-associated hepatitis in Labrador retrievers. *Vet. Pathol.* 46 (3): 484–490.

16 Jaimie, M., Strickland, J.M., Buchweitz, J.P. et al. (2018). Hepatic copper concentrations in 546 dogs (1982–2015). *J. Vet. Intern. Med.* 32 (6): 1943–1950.

17 Spee, B., Arends, B., van den Ingh, T.S. et al. (2006). Copper metabolism and oxidative stress in chronic inflammatory and cholestatic liver diseases in dogs. *J. Vet. Intern. Med.* 20 (5): 1085–1092.

18 Azumi, N. (1982). Copper and liver injury – experimental studies on the dogs with biliary obstruction and copper loading. *Hokkaido Igaky Zasshi* 57 (3): 331–349.

19 Van den Ingh, T.S.G.A.M., van Winkle, T., Cullen, J.M. et al. (2006). Morphological classification of parenchymal disorders of the canine and feline liver – hepatocellular death, hepatitis and cirrhosis. In: *Standard for Clinical and Histological Diagnosis of Canine and Feline Liver Disease* (ed. WSAVA Liver Standardization Group), 85–101. St Louis, MO: Saunders.

20 Russell Moore, A., Medrano, E., Coffey, E., and Powers, B. (2019). Clinicopathological correlation and prevalence of increased copper in canine hepatic cytology. *J. Am. Anim. Hosp. Assoc.* 55 (1): 8–13.

21 Moore, A.R., Coffey, E., and Hamar, D. (2016). Diagnostic accuracy of Wright-Giemsa and rhodanine stain protocols for detection and semi-quantitative grading of copper in canine liver aspirates. *Vet. Clin. Pathol.* 45 (4): 689–697.

22 Salaspuro, M. and Sipponen, P. (1976). Demonstration of an intracellular copper-binding protein by orcein staining in long-standing cholestatic liver diseases. *Gut* 17 (10): 787–790.

23 Hultgren, B.D., Stevens, J.B., and Hardy, R.M. (1986). Inherited, chronic, progressive hepatic degeneration in Bedlington terriers with increased liver copper concentrations: clinical and pathologic observations and comparison with other copper-associated liver diseases. *Am. J. Vet. Res.* 47 (2): 365–377.

24 Van den Ingh, T.S.G.A.M., Rothuizen, J., and Meyer, H.P. (1995). Circulatory disorders of the liver in dogs and cats. *Vet. Q.* 17 (2): 70–76.

25 Rollois, M., Ruel, Y., and Besso, J.G. (2003). Passive liver congestion associated with caudal vena caval compression due to oesophageal leiomyoma. *J. Small Anim. Pract.* 44 (10): 460–463.

26 Garden, O.A., Kidd, L., Mexas, A.M. et al. (2019). ACVIM consensus statement on the diagnosis of immune-mediated hemolytic anemia in dogs and cats. *J. Vet. Intern. Med.* 33 (2): 313–334.

27 Gultekin, G.I., Raj, K., Foureman, P. et al. (2012). Erythrocytic pyruvate kinase mutations causing hemolytic anemia, osteosclerosis, and secondary hemochromatosis in dogs. *J. Vet. Intern. Med.* 26 (4): 935–944.

28 Sprague, W.S., Hackett, T.B., Johnson, J.S. et al. (2003). Hemochromatosis secondary to repeated blood transfusions in a dog. *Vet. Pathol.* 40 (3): 334–337.

29 Greijdanus-van der Putten, S.W.M., van Esch, E., Kamerman, J. et al. (2005). Drug-induced protoporphyria in beagle dogs. *Toxicol. Pathol.* 33 (6): 720–725.

30 Veldhuis Kroeze, E.J.B., Zentek, J., Edixhoven-Bosdijk, A. et al. (2006). Transient erythropoietic protoporphyria associated with chronic hepatitis and cirrhosis in a cohort of German shepherd dogs. *Vet. Rec.* 158 (4): 120–124.

31 Kunz, B.C., Center, S.A., Randolph, J.F. et al. (2020). Congenital erythropoietic protoporphyria and protoporphyric hepatopathy in a dog. *J. Am. Vet. Med. Assoc.* 257 (11): 1148–1156.

32 Hetz, C. (2012). The unfolded protein response: controlling cell fate decisions under ER stress and beyond. *Nat. Rev. Mol. Cell Biol.* 13 (2): 89–102.

33 Masserdotti, C., Rossetti, E., de Lorenzi, D. et al. (2014). Characterization of cytoplasmic hyaline bodies in a hepatocellular carcinoma of a dog. *Res. Vet. Sci.* 96 (1): 143–146.

34 Kurtovich, E. and Limaiem, F. (2022). Mallory bodies. www.ncbi.nlm.nih.gov/ books/NBK545300/ StatPearl Publishing, September, 12, 2022.

35 Johnson, A.M. (2006). Amino acids, peptides and proteins. In: *Tietz Textbook of Clinical Chemistry and Molecular Diagnostics* (ed. C.A. Burtis, E.R. Ashwood, and D.E. Bruns), 550–551. St Louis, MO: Elsevier Saunders.

36 Takeda, M. (1983). *Atlas of Diagnostic Gastrointestinal Cytology.* Tokyo, Japan: Igaku-Shoin.

37 Sevelius, E., Andersson, M., and Jönsson, L. (1994). Hepatic accumulation of alpha-1-antitrypsin in chronic liver disease in the dog. *J. Comp. Pathol.* 111 (4): 401–412.

38 Van Winkle, T., Cullen, J.M., van den Ingh, T.S.G.A.M. et al. (2006). Morphological classification of parenchymal disorders of the canine and feline liver – hepatic abcesses and granulomas, hepatic metabolic storage disorders and miscellaneous conditions. In: *Standard for Clinical and Histological Diagnosis of Canine and Feline Liver Disease* (ed. WSAVA Liver Standardization Group), 103–116. St Louis, MO: Saunders.

39 Haskins, M.E., Otis, E.J., Hayden, J.E. et al. (1992). Hepatic storage of glycosaminoglycans in feline and canine models of mucopolysaccharidoses I, VI, and VII. *Vet. Pathol.* 29 (2): 112–119.

40 Center, S.A., Guida, L., Zanelli, M.J. et al. (1993). Ultrastructural hepatocellular features associated with severe hepatic lipidosis in cats. *Am. J. Vet. Res.* 54 (5): 724–731.

41 Rothuizen, J., van den Brom, W.E., and Fevery, J. (1992). The origins and kinetics of bilirubin in dogs with hepatobiliary and haemolytic diseases. *J. Hepatol.* 15 (1–2): 17–24.

42 DiBartola, S.P. and Benson, M.D. (1989). The pathogenesis of reactive systemic amyloidosis. *J. Vet. Intern. Med.* 3 (1): 31–41.

43 Beatty, J.A., Barrs, V.R., Martin, P.A. et al. (2002). Spontaneous hepatic rupture in six cats with systemic amyloidosis. *J. Small Anim. Pract.* 43 (8): 355–363.

44 Neo-Suzuki, S., Mineshige, T., Kamiie, J. et al. (2017). Hepatic AA amyloidosis in a cat: cytologic and histologic identification of AA amyloid in macrophages. *Vet. Clin. Pathol.* 46 (2): 331–336.

45 Carothers, M.A., Johnson, G.C., DiBartola, S.P. et al. (1989). Extramedullary plasmacytoma and immunoglobulin-associated amyloidosis in a cat. *J. Am. Vet. Med. Assoc.* 195 (11): 1593–1597.

5

Irreversible Hepatocellular Damage

Some pathological conditions – especially extreme hypoxia and the action of toxic molecules or etiological agents – can result in damage so severe as to directly cause the death of the hepatocyte [1]. The death of the hepatocyte can occur as necrosis or apoptosis. The belief that the prevalence of necrosis or apoptosis is a direct consequence of the nature, extent, and duration of a given primary cause is widely acknowledged [2].

5.1 Necrosis

Cytomorphology: cytoplasm shows a blurred profile, frequent tendency to disintegrate, irregular granular appearance, basophilic or grayish color (Figure 5.1); shrinkage of the nucleus, that frequently appears evanescent or completely disintegrated (Figures 5.2 and 5.3); groups of hepatocytes affected by necrosis may merge or be replaced by variably basophilic material in large aggregates (Figures 5.4 and 5.5), represented by cellular necrotic debris; frequent association with inflammatory cells, mostly neutrophilic granulocytes or macrophages (Figure 5.6).

In coagulative necrosis, the affected cells maintain a vaguely normal round shape although, because of cytoplasmic and membranous protein denaturation and swelling of cytoplasm, hepatocytes appear pale and indistinct; nuclear pycnosis or karyolysis leading to shrinkage or disintegration of the nucleus are common. In contrast, in "liquefactive" or "lithic" necrosis, the cause of hepatocyte death leads to complete loss of all morphological features.

From a cytological point of view, distinction between the two types of necrosis is not important, nor is it feasible. The cells sampled from areas affected by coagulative necrosis may be recognized by their irregularly round profile and loss

Canine and Feline Liver Cytology, First Edition. Carlo Masserdotti.
© 2024 John Wiley & Sons, Inc. Published 2024 by John Wiley & Sons, Inc.

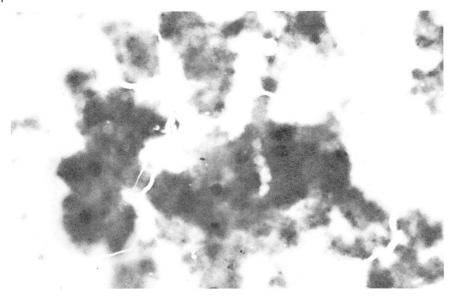

Figure 5.1   Liver, necrosis, FNCS, dog. In colliquative necrosis, although the outline of the cytoplasm and the presence of pyknotic nuclei are recognizable, the cells look completely disarranged (MGG, 100×).

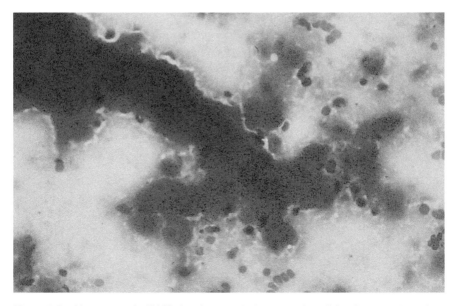

Figure 5.2   Liver, necrosis, FNCS, dog. In coagulative necrosis, cell borders are blurred and evanescent, nuclei are shrunken and disaggregated, but epithelial cells are still recognizable (MGG, 100×).

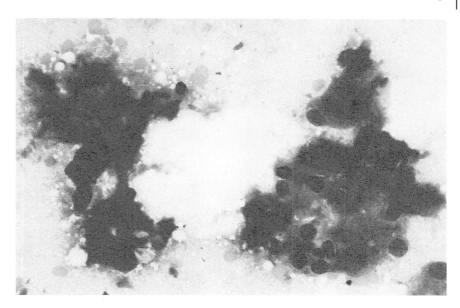

Figure 5.3 Liver, necrosis and cholestasis, FNCS, dog. Note the difference between live hepatocytes, on the right, crossed by biliary casts, and necrotic cells on the left (MGG, 100×).

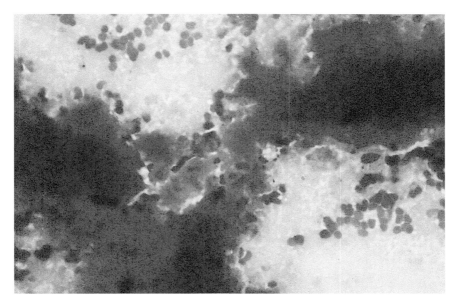

Figure 5.4 Liver, necrosis, FNCS, dog. In coagulative necrosis, although living cells are still recognizable, dead hepatocytes accumulate in large basophilic clumps (MGG, 100×).

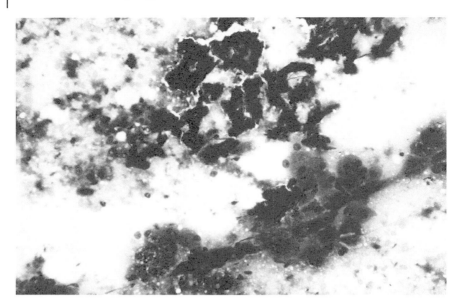

Figure 5.5 Liver, necrosis, FNCS, dog. Hepatocytes (bottom right) surrounded by large clumps of necrotic material (MGG, 100×).

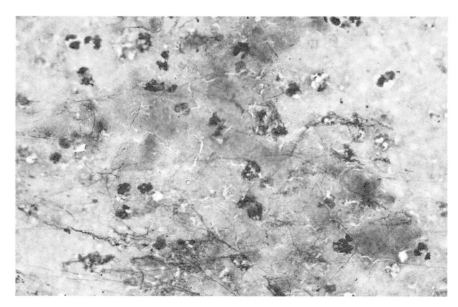

Figure 5.6 Liver, necrosis, FNCS, dog. Large amounts of necrotic material, represented by gray-bluish cellular bodies, associated with scattered degenerate neutrophilic granulocytes (MGG, 100×).

of cytoplasmic and nuclear details; however, the trauma caused by sampling and preparation can lead to disruption of the weak bodies of dead cells and distribution, on the slide, of irregularly dispersed necrotic material, indistinguishable from colliquative necrosis. The necrotic material appears granular or basophilic, as dispersed debris or aggregated in clumps, sometimes associated with groups of normal or variably damaged hepatocytes. This depends on the action and extent of the necrotizing event.

Learning to distinguish necrotic hepatocytes is crucial as morphological analysis is key to diagnosis and prognosis and, above all, to distinguish them from morphologically similar events such as the accumulation of platelet aggregates, proteinaceous debris or gel used for ultrasonographic investigation. When necrosis is detected cytologically, a complete and detailed evaluation of the smears must be carried out, looking for suppurative inflammation, bacterial phagocytosis or the presence of neoplastic cells.

These processes are generally the causes of the most extensive irreversible damage and can underlie the loss of hepatocytes in very large areas of the parenchyma – sometimes with alterations detectable by ultrasonographic or tomographic examination – and, in more extreme cases, fatal damage to the parenchyma.

In *coagulative* necrosis, denaturation of cytoplasmic proteins leads to cell death; denaturation of cytoplasmic and membrane proteins, swelling of cells, pycnosis or nuclear karyolysis are frequent features, although the cells maintain their round shape unaltered.

In *liquefactive* or *lytic* necrosis, which occurs in the presence of extensive destruction of hepatocytes with swelling and disintegration of the cytoplasm, the shape and profile of the hepatocytes are completely lost. In irreversible hepatocellular damage, the membrane loses its ability to control the normal gradients of ions and metabolites between the cytoplasm and the extracellular space. As necrosis develops, all cytoplasmic constituents are irreparably damaged and released. The damage induced by primary causes can lead to cell death through various mechanisms, including altered membrane permeability leading to accumulation of Ca^{2+} ions in the cytosol and mitochondria, as well as termination of nucleic acid or protein synthesis – a consequence of decreased ATP production or damage to the membranes [3]. In these cases, leakage of the hepatic enzymes ALT and AST (an indirect biochemical indication of hepatocellular damage) is mediated by this devastating mechanism; it is completely different from the mechanism that leads to nonspecific and reversible damage, which is generally mediated by the detachment of cytoplasmic vesicles from structurally intact cells ("blebbing") [4].

Necrotic processes can involve single cells or, more frequently, extend to large areas of the parenchyma. Frequently, the presence of irregularly distributed and multifocal areas of necrosis in the parenchyma is a consequence of gastrointestinal-derived, embolic septic events. In contrast, the presence of zonal or more extensive necrosis is generally caused by hypoxic or toxic damage [5]; when the damage is localized within the centrilobular area, hypoxia and intoxication are generally deemed as the most likely causes but when it is localized within the periportal area, infection becomes much more likely.

The causes of zonal damage have been investigated at length in numerous studies and histopathological evaluations but this is beyond the scope of this book. Very frequently, the necrosis of either single or small groups of cells, especially if mediated by causes that have already ceased, is characterized by minimal morphological phenomena. For example, when focal necrosis occurs, Kupffer cells, sometimes together with neutrophils and lymphocytes, remove the necrotic cellular material and form small aggregates called lipogranulomas – discussed in Chapter 6 on inflammatory diseases [6]. In confluent and bridging necrosis, large groups of dead hepatocytes with zonal distribution, that can occur in centrilobular, midzonal and periportal areas, are generally evident. In massive necrosis, extensive and diffuse panlobar or multilobar death takes place; in that instance, complete disarrangement of the anatomical distribution of liver architecture occurs.

The most frequent causes of hepatocellular necrosis include severe acute hypoxia [7], as in the course of immune-mediated hemolytic anemia [8]; food poisonings are also described, including the consumption of poisonous mushrooms (well known in human medicine), such as *Amanita phalloides* [9] or aflatoxins. The most frequent toxic cause is the administration of pharmacological molecules (acetaminophen, halothane, benzodiazepines, sulfonamide-trimethoprim association, carprofen and amiodarone, phenobarbital), as well as several others that are normally administered to the dog and cat. Normal biochemical transformation or biotransformation intended to transform lipophilic molecules into water-soluble molecules for excretion into the bile is carried out by the centrilobular hepatocytes. Potentially harmless molecules are biotransformed into highly reactive metabolites intended to be conjugated to polar molecules for excretion. In certain cases of overdose or insufficient polar molecules such as glutathione, the reactive forms bind to cellular enzymes or subcellular structural elements in the centrilobular hepatocyte [10].

Alternatively, the invasion may be blood based, more specifically when the portal blood carries bacteria from the intestine to the sinusoids: here, in the presence of multifocal areas affected by preexisting necrosis, with loss of both mechanical barriers and cellular immune control, bacteria can invade the parenchyma and lead to necrotic damage.

It should always be borne in mind that although morphological features of necrosis are easily detectable, cytology is never able to establish where the damage is located and therefore, in some cases, histology is necessary to acquire further information.

5.2   Apoptosis

Cytomorphology: decreased size of cytoplasm, round to polygonal shape, eosinophilic and homogeneous content (Figure 5.7); nucleus is pyknotic, small in size,
with dense, homogeneous chromatin (Figure 5.8); mainly affecting single and
sporadic hepatocytes, wedged between unaffected hepatocytes (Figure 5.9);
inflammation and fibrosis features may be present (Figure 5.10).

Apoptosis is the programmed death of cells, mediated by the action of cytoplasmic caspases, enzymes that induce shrinkage of the cytoplasm and of the
nucleus, which acquires a typically pyknotic compact and hyperchromatic
appearance. Although this type of cell death is considered to be physiological in
some circumstances, thus sporadic and affecting exclusively cells that have
reached the end of their natural life, apoptosis may also be caused by pathological conditions that activate the same mechanisms, though on a higher number of
cells than normal. According to the literature on hepatic pathology [1], apoptosis
of single hepatocytes is mostly observed during chronic hepatitis, a prolonged
inflammatory event determined by multifactorial causes that are often difficult
to recognize (about 30% caused by copper in dogs). If causes are not removed,
chronic hepatitis is an irreversible pathological process that includes variable

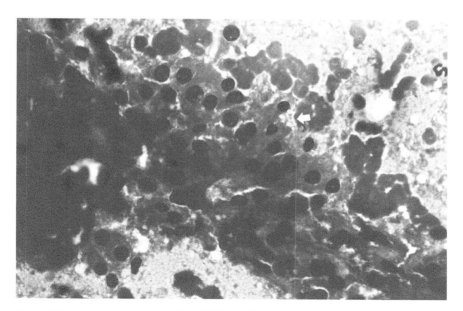

Figure 5.7   Liver, aspecific hepatitis, FNCS, dog. Two apoptotic hepatocytes (white arrow),
indicated by eosinophilic cytoplasm and shrunken, hyperchromatic nuclei (MGG, 100×).

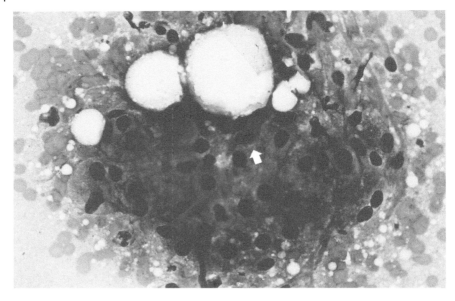

Figure 5.8 Liver, aspecific hepatitis, FNCS, dog. An apoptotic hepatocyte (white arrow) among living cells; notice the small size, irregular shape, eosinophilic cytoplasm, and hyperchromatic nucleus (MGG, 100×).

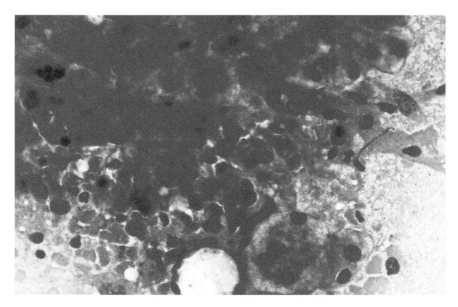

Figure 5.9 Liver, chronic hepatitis, FNCS, dog. Apoptotic hepatocytes may be observed in aggregates of living hepatocytes (MGG, 100×).

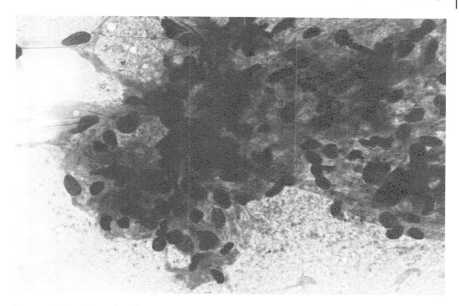

Figure 5.10 Liver, chronic hepatitis, FNCS, dog. Apoptotic hepatocytes may be observed sometimes close to bundles of fibrillary material and spindle cells in fibrosis (MGG, 100×).

extension of portal fibrosis, sometimes porto-portal or porto-central, with periportal accumulation of inflammatory elements and apoptotic events affecting mostly periportal hepatocytes.

Cytological recognition of apoptotic cells is easier when hepatocytes are in bidimensional sheets, while it is difficult in tridimensional aggregates. Apoptotic cells must be morphologically differentiated from artifactually disrupted hepatocytes, from mast cells and from small platelet aggregates. Apoptosis is a pathological phenomenon that is rarely observed by cytology; indeed, in my experience, it is quite difficult to detect as the apoptotic cell (generally surrounded by normal hepatocytes or affected by nonspecific damage) is smaller and features intensely eosinophilic cytoplasm and a pyknotic nucleus. Despite the association of apoptosis with chronic hepatitis, the presence of apoptotic cells was not evaluated in one study on the cytological features of hepatic fibrosis [11].

When apoptotic cells are detected, it is advisable to investigate the rest of the sample for possible presence of fibrotic events (see Chapter 8), association with reversible hepatocellular damage, and inflammatory processes. If the morphological features are compatible with the clinical and anamnestic data, as well as with the laboratory diagnostics data and the results of ultrasonographic imaging of the parenchyma, chronic hepatitis may be a plausible conclusion, but this must be confirmed by histopathological investigation.

The hepatocyte undergoes programmed death involving mostly single cells, with cell shrinkage and fragmentation. Phagocytosis is enhanced by biochemical changes in the cell membranes and fragments are ingested by Kupffer cells, sometimes from hepatocytes. Piecemeal necrosis, which occurs when hepatocytes of the limiting plate are damaged by surrounding inflammatory cells, is mostly characterized by apoptosis [1]. This is a process that is generally characterized by the death of single cells and is never extensive or massive.

5.3   Key Points

- Necrosis represents a wide, destructive injury to hepatocytes; when present, always consider severe hypoxia, toxicity, infective diseases, mostly bacterial, or associated neoplastic diseases.
- Apoptosis is programmed cell death, that occurs as single-cell phenomenon; its recognition is difficult, to be distinguished by artifactual shrinkage of the cell, by normal hepatic mast cells and by small platelet aggregates; when present, look for fibrosis or others features of chronic inflammation.

References

1 Van den Ingh, T.S.G.A.M., van Winkle, T., Cullen, J.M. et al. (2006). Morphological classification of parenchymal disorders of the canine and feline liver – hepatocellular death, hepatitis and cirrhosis. In: *Standard for Clinical and Histological Diagnosis of Canine and Feline Liver Disease* (ed. WSAVA Liver Standardization Group), 85–101. St Louis, MO: Saunders.

2 Kaplowitz, N. (2002). Biochemical and cellular mechanism of toxic liver injury. *Semin. Liver Dis.* 22: 137–144.

3 Decker, K. (1993). Mechanism and mediators in hepatic necrosis. *Gastroenterol. Jpn.* 28 (Suppl. 4): 20–25.

4 Stockham, S.L. and Scott, M.A. (2008). Enzymes. In: *Fundamentals of Veterinary Clinical Pathology*, IIe, 640–650. Ames, IO: Blackwell Publishing.

5 Hayes, M.A. (2004). Pathophysiology of the liver. In: *Veterinary Pathophysiology* (ed. R.H. Dunlop and C.H. Malbert), 392–393. Ames, IA: Blackwell Publishing.

6 Van Winkle, T., Cullen, J.M., van den Ingh, T.S.G.A.M. et al. (2006). Morphological classification of parenchymal disorders of the canine and feline liver – hepatic abcesses and granulomas, hepatic metabolic storage disorders and miscellaneous conditions. In: *Standard for Clinical and Histological Diagnosis of Canine and Feline Liver Disease* (ed. WSAVA Liver Standardization Group), 103–116. St Louis, MO: Saunders.

7 Smith, M.K. and Mooney, D.J. (2007). Hypoxia leads to necrotic hepatocyte death. *J. Biomed. Mater. Res. A* 80 (3): 520–529.

8 McManus, P.M. and Craig, L.E. (2001). Correlation between leukocytosis and necropsy findings in dogs with immune-mediated hemolytic anemia: 34 cases (1994–1999). *J. Am. Vet. Med. Assoc.* 218 (8): 1308–1313.

9 Watanabe, S. and Philips, M.J. (1986). Acute phalloidin toxicity in living hepatocytes. Evidence for a possible disturbance in membrane flow and for multiple function for actin in the liver cell. *Am. J. Pathol.* 122: 101–111.

10 Cullen, J.M. (2005). Mechanistic classification of liver injury. *Toxicol. Pathol.* 33: 6–8.

11 Masserdotti, C. and Bertazzolo, W. (2016). Cytologic features of hepatic fibrosis in dogs: a retrospective study on 22 cases. *Vet. Clin. Pathol.* 45: 361–367.

6

Inflammation

This area of cytology is certainly easy, enjoyable, and rewarding when dealing with diseases affecting the skin, lungs, prostate, and many other anatomical areas; however, when it comes to the liver, it turns into a minefield. A misstep could mean producing results that confuse or even mislead the clinician. Cytology frequently provides valuable information, especially related to the presence or the role of etiological agents as the cause of an inflammatory process. However, cytology loses its effectiveness when, despite the presence of an inflammatory process localized in the parenchyma, no etiological agents are detected. More specifically, the morphological data become "blurred," which often makes histopathological evaluation necessary to arrive at a diagnosis.

Discrepancies in the diagnostic value of cytology in the identification of hepatitis are common. Wang et al. found that hepatitis was correctly identified on cytology in five of 20 dogs and three of 11 cats [1]. Weiss found the sensitivity and specificity of nonstandardized subjective cytological assessments for predicting a histopathological diagnosis of hepatitis to be 93% and 96%, respectively [2].

The main reason for these discrepancies is that criteria for cytological diagnosis of hepatitis are subjective. Evidence of inflammation in the liver acquires meaning only when the peculiar microanatomy of this organ is considered, which normally makes histopathological investigation necessary. However, often the cause of an acute or chronic hepatic inflammation cannot easily be recognized even by histopathology and an etiological diagnosis frequently remains undetermined. Nevertheless, a cytologically nonspecific inflammatory finding may acquire diagnostic power when compared with the histological pattern: lobular location (periportal, midzonal or centrilobular); fibrosis (or elements suggesting its imminent onset); distribution and association with hepatocellular damage; possible evidence of vascular alterations or damage to the biliary structures. For example, if the inflammation is concentrated in the periportal area, the most likely diseases

Canine and Feline Liver Cytology, First Edition. Carlo Masserdotti.
© 2024 John Wiley & Sons, Inc. Published 2024 by John Wiley & Sons, Inc.

are either, on rare occasions, toxic based or bacterial/viral etiological borne (via portal blood or due to infection of the ascending bile ducts). Alternatively, if the inflammation is detected near or in the bile ducts, cholangitis or cholangio-hepatitis, when both bile ducts and adjacent hepatocytes are affected, either infectious or toxic, are most likely. Even if the liver sample features obvious and repeatable inflammation, recognizing the primary cause(s) is normally impossible. In addition, in the course of most pathological conditions, the liver responds with a rather peculiar inflammatory pattern, especially if compared to those detected in other organs. For example, acute hepatitis is characterized by inflammatory infiltrate, including hepatocellular apoptosis, necrosis (in proportion with the causes) and, in some cases, regeneration [3]. Unless an inflammatory process is detected, these morphological features may be difficult (if not impossible) to detect in a cytological sample, especially if they are present in only small amounts.

Chronic hepatitis is characterized by the presence of fibrosis when detected in addition to inflammation, apoptosis, and necrosis [3]. This can be ascertained by cytological investigation (more information in Chapter 8) but the role, severity, and distribution of inflammation and fibrosis (all necessary for a diagnosis) can only be fully assessed by histological investigation. Consequently, unlike the situation in other organs, the cytologist must always bear in mind that detecting neutrophilic granulocytes, lymphocytes, and macrophages dispersed among the hepatocytes of a cytological sample is not enough to diagnose a suppurative, lymphocytic or granulomatous hepatitis. This information is of little specific meaning in the absence of information relating to the other criteria concerning the diagnosis of inflammation and, moreover, a histological examination.

Indeed, the presence of numerous leukocytes in a hepatic cytological sample can be a marker of hepatic inflammation, but it should be noted that there are differential causes for this and some are not related to liver inflammation. The first alternative possibility is contamination by blood, especially when hematological examination of the peripheral blood indicates a leukocytosis. The blood sampled by a hepatic needle aspirate may contain hepatic cells, but it may also contain a sufficient number of leukocytes to suggest a potential inflammation. A differential count between the leukocyte concentration of the peripheral blood and that of the blood found in the liver sample is therefore strongly advised. Although this approach has not been confirmed by relevant studies, it is logical to suggest that if the differential count of the blood leukocytes is similar to that of the liver sample, the presence of leukocytes, even in large numbers, is very likely to be caused by contamination of the blood sample. Differential counting as an empirical method to exclude blood as the source of the neutrophils is a quite complex procedure to perform.

In addition to inflammation, which may lead to an increase in the number of leukocytes in a hepatic cytological sample, extramedullary hematopoiesis may also suggest a possible inflammatory role of the leukocytes. However, the evidence of several immature forms reduces the possibility of misinterpretation. Although it may be considered normal, especially in young animals (see Chapter 2), extramedullary granulocytic hematopoiesis may develop within the connective tissue surrounding the portal tracts or centrilobular vessels, during septic bacterial diseases, some chronic injuries, and within the parenchyma of primary hepatocellular neoplasms. Extramedullary myelopoiesis is also present in dogs with steroid-induced hepatopathy and sometimes associated with systemic acute or chronic inflammatory conditions.

After downplaying the role of cytology in assessing inflammatory liver diseases, I will admit that, in some scenarios, cytology may be sufficient to recognize the causes of a condition and therefore produce a diagnosis. To simplify the discussion on inflammatory processes, the role of each inflammatory population will be discussed in the following sections.

6.1 Presence of Neutrophilic Granulocytes

Cytomorphology: variable number of well-differentiated or degenerate neutrophilic granulocytes on the background or wedged between hepatocytes (Figure 6.1); in samples from hepatic abscesses, the number of neutrophils is generally very high

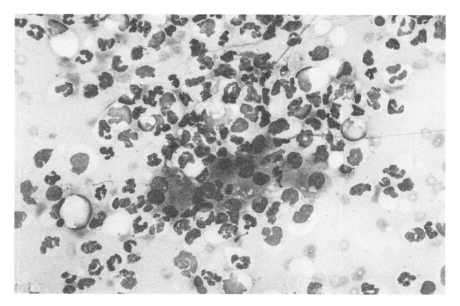

Figure 6.1 Liver, septic suppurative hepatitis, FNCS, dog. Many well-preserved or karyolytic neutrophilic granulocytes that surround and infiltrate a small aggregate of hepatocytes. Dog, acute suppurative hepatitis (MGG, 100×).

and may overwhelm the number of hepatocytes; phagocytosis of bacteria in septic inflammation is possible (Figures 6.2 and 6.3); association with macrophages or lymphoplasma cells is frequent in cases of chronic inflammatory conditions (Figure 6.4); reversible or irreversible damage of hepatocytes is frequently observed (Figure 6.5); association with other pathological conditions, like cholestasis or fibrosis, is possible (Figure 6.6).

The presence and number of neutrophilic granulocytes in a cytological sample from the liver must be carefully evaluated and interpreted (Table 6.1); indeed, when they are dispersed on a bloody background and do not feature degenerative aspects, blood contamination tends to be more likely (Figure 6.7). In this case, as previously stated, comparison with the leukogram should be useful. There are few studies evaluating the correlation between neutrophil count and a histopathological diagnosis of hepatitis. Recently, a study was conducted to evaluate whether the number of neutrophils seen on cytology smears could be used as a marker of hepatitis. Results suggest that identification of ≥6 neutrophils/200 hepatocytes is highly suggestive of hepatitis, independent of the primary process [4]. Another condition that must be excluded is myelopoiesis, which can occur in dogs with steroid-induced hepatopathy or extrahepatic inflammations; in these cases, the presence of myelocytes or band granulocytes is the diagnostic key to differentiate myelopoiesis from true inflammation (Figure 6.8).

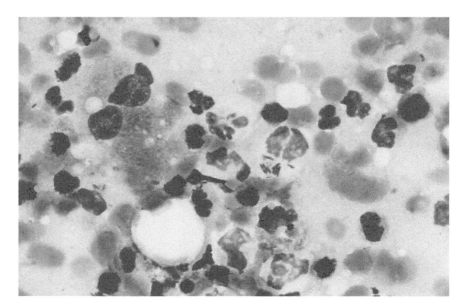

Figure 6.2 Liver, septic suppurative hepatitis, FNCS, dog. Neutrophilic phagocytosis of rod-shaped bacteria. Dog, septic suppurative hepatitis (MGG, 100×).

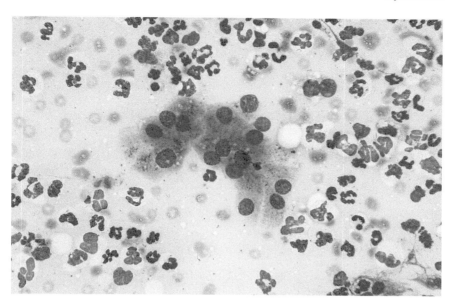

Figure 6.3 Liver, septic suppurative hepatitis, FNCS, dog. Neutrophilic phagocytosis of filamentous bacteria. Dog, septic suppurative hepatitis (MGG, 100×).

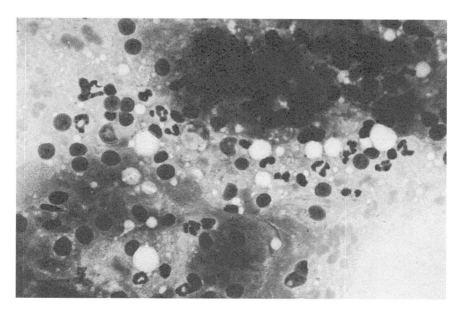

Figure 6.4 Liver, chronic aspecific hepatitis, FNCS, dog. Presence of neutrophils with lymphocytes and macrophages in mixed, chronic inflammation (MGG, 100×).

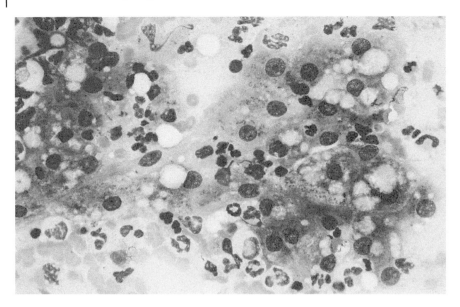

Figure 6.5 Liver, acute suppurative hepatitis, FNCS, dog. Degenerative changes of hepatocytes with mixed, mostly neutrophilic inflammation (MGG, 100×).

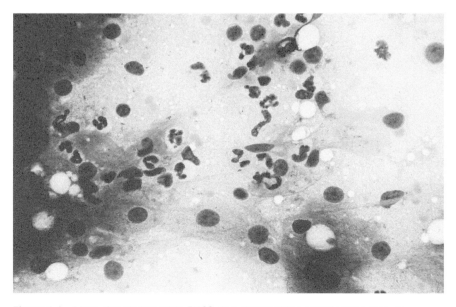

Figure 6.6 Liver, chronic hepatitis, FNCS, dog. Neutrophilic granulocytes close to bundles of collagen (MGG, 100×).

Table 6.1   Common causes of suppurative inflammation.

Acute bacterial hepatitis or cholangitis

Hepatic abscesses

Viral diseases (FIP in cats; canine adenovirus-1 in dogs)

Neoplasia

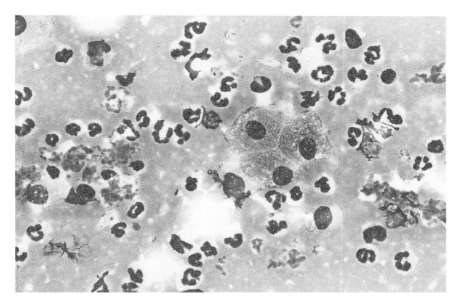

Figure 6.7   Normal liver, staging of lymphoma, FNCS, dog. Presence of many neutrophils, together with lymphocytes and platelet aggregates, mostly present on the border of the smear, indicate blood contamination rather than true inflammation (MGG, 100×).

However, the criteria I use to corroborate a suppurative inflammatory process are different. Generally, one can subjectively evaluate the number of neutrophils, considering it increased when approximately 2–3 neutrophils are present together with hepatocytes in most high-power fields or when dominating the number of total nucleated cells. The morphological evaluation of neutrophils is mandatory, as the presence of karyolysis or karyopyknosis is a more reliable marker of an inflammatory process – possibly to be compared with other parameters of inflammation, including hyperthermia, the leukocyte concentration, the morphological aspects of circulating neutrophilic granulocytes and the concentration of the PCR.

One of the most effective morphological criteria indicating an inflammatory role for neutrophilic granulocytes is their location: clustered (Figure 6.9) or

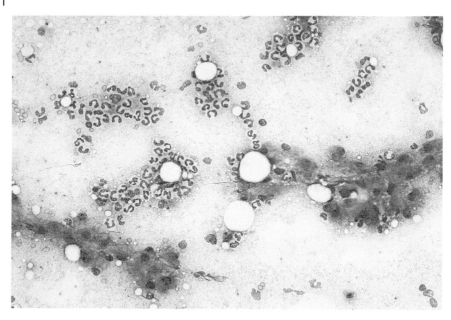

Figure 6.8 Liver, extramedullary myelopoiesis, FNCS, dog. Presence of band neutrophils indicates extramedullary hematopoiesis rather than inflammation; the sample was obtained during an ultrasonographic diagnosis of pyometra (MGG, 100×).

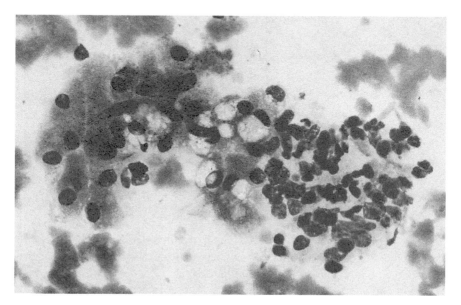

Figure 6.9 Liver, acute suppurative hepatitis, FNCS, dog. Clustering of degenerate neutrophils around the hepatocytes (MGG, 100×).

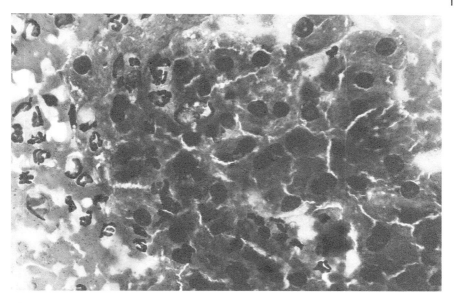

Figure 6.10 Liver, suppurative hepatitis, FNCS, dog. Notice the distribution of neutrophils into the epithelial aggregate, mostly wedged among hepatocytes (MGG, 100×).

wedged (Figure 6.10) rather than accumulated at the edges of the hepatocyte aggregates or dispersed on the bottom.

Even if all the aforesaid features of suppurative inflammation are detected, it is important to remember that the findings are frequently nonspecific and that comparison with the histological investigation is always necessary, especially to identify the location of the inflammatory process within the hepatic lobule.

In the suppurative hepatitis cases I have encountered in my practice, the cyto-morphological findings included an extremely high neutrophil/hepatocyte ratio, the presence of neutrophilic degeneration, necrotic material dispersed on the background and, in some cases, evidence of bacterial phagocytosis. Suppurative hepatitis may follow many primary causes, which generally lead to cholangitis, acute or chronic hepatitis, sometimes related to secondary bacterial infection of the parenchyma. Suppurative hepatitis may sometimes be due to an abscess (ultrasound investigation for corroboration is helpful), that is most often caused by bacterial infections that reach the parenchyma through the portal vein, ascending the biliary ducts or by direct traumatic penetration of the liver; furthermore, in very young animals, they may also develop as a result of infections coming from the umbilical vein. Another possible cause of abscesses (sometimes large) is bacterial contamination of necrotic or hemorrhagic areas within primary or metastatic neoplasms.

A variable number (from 1–5 cells/HPF to 5–10 cells/HPF) of well-preserved or degenerate neutrophils may be observed in cases of acute or chronic cholestasis and of acute or chronic cholangitis [5].

A moderate to large amount of well-preserved neutrophils, together with many macrophages, sometimes with lymphocytes and plasma cells (Figure 6.11), are present in the liver of cats affected by feline infectious peritonitis (FIP) [6, 7]. The inflammatory cells sometimes aggregate in cohesive groups around the hepato-cytes (Figure 6.12). Although the cytological features are nonspecific, FIP should be considered among the differential diagnoses when a mixed inflammation is observed in a cytological sample of liver from a cat. This is supported by a study which revealed that the presence of mixed inflammatory cells was consistent with FIP in 14/22 cases from fine needle aspirates of the liver [8].

Although rare, neutrophils in the liver have also been described in association with a Sarcocystidae infection [9].

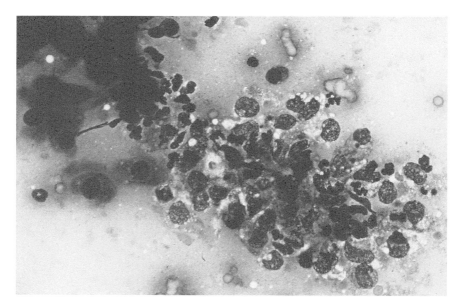

Figure 6.11 Liver, FIP, FNCS, cat. Aggregate of macrophages, lymphocytes, and neutrophils in a cat with FIP infection (MGG, 100×).

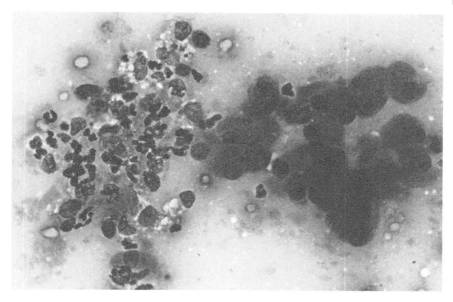

Figure 6.12 Liver, FIP, FNCS, cat. Well-preserved neutrophils and macrophages aggregate around a cluster of normal hepatocytes, in a cat with FIP infection (MGG, 100×).

6.2 Presence of Eosinophilic Granulocytes

Cytomorphology: increased number of eosinophilic granulocytes scattered on the background, around hepatocyte aggregates (Figure 6.13), sometimes wedged between hepatocytes (Figure 6.14); reversible damage of hepatocytes is possible; association with other inflammatory populations is sometime observed.

As previously discussed, in order to correctly identify true inflammation, comparison of the number of eosinophils in liver aspirates with their percentage in peripheral blood is mandatory in the exclusion of blood contamination. The cytological cases in which the number of eosinophilic granulocytes is sufficient to indicate an inflammatory role are very rare indeed (Table 6.2). In years of practice, I was lucky enough to observe a handful of cases. Eosinophils may be more common in young animals, possibly due to nematode, cestode or trematode larval migration, and I considered generating an inflammatory response or hypersensitivity conditions. However, this is rarely confirmed by histopathological investigation. Consequently, I have never gained sufficient experience to be able to comment on the causes which, according to the literature, are hypereosinophilic

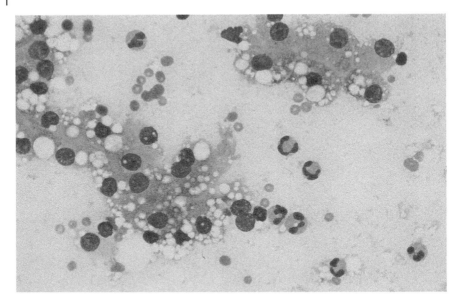

Figure 6.13   Liver, eosinophilic hepatitis of unknown cause, FNCS, dog. Many eosinophilic granulocytes dispersed around hepatocytes (MGG, 100×).

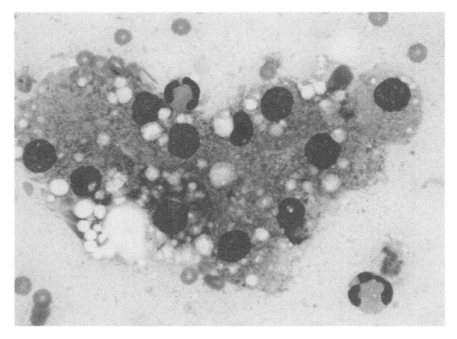

Figure 6.14   Liver, eosinophilic hepatitis of unknown cause, FNCS, dog. Eosinophils are sometimes wedged among hepatocytes (MGG, 100×).

Table 6.2   Common causes of eosinophilic inflammation.

Adverse drug reaction

Parasites

syndrome, forms of nonspecific reactive hepatitis, and adverse drug reactions [3].
An inflammatory eosinophilic component associated with neutrophilic granulocytes and lymphocytes was described in a dog with Sarcoystidae hepatitis [10].

6.3   Presence of Lymphocytes and Plasma Cells

Cytomorphology: polymorphic population of small to intermediate, sometimes
large lymphoid cells, scattered on the background, together with a variable number of plasma cells, sometimes crowded around the hepatocyte clusters
(Figures 6.15 and 6.16); association with other inflammatory cells is possible
(Figure 6.17); hepatocellular damage (Figure 6.18), fibrosis (Figure 6.19) or necrosis are possible; association with biliary cells is also possible.

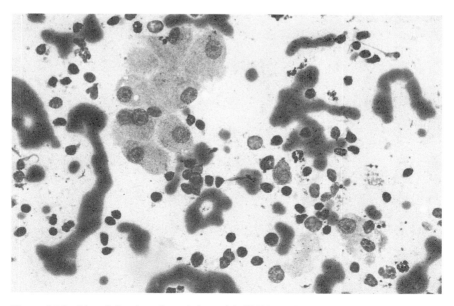

Figure 6.15   Liver, feline lymphocytic hepatitis, FNCS, cat. Polymorphic lymphocytes are
scattered among hepatocytes (MGG, 100×).

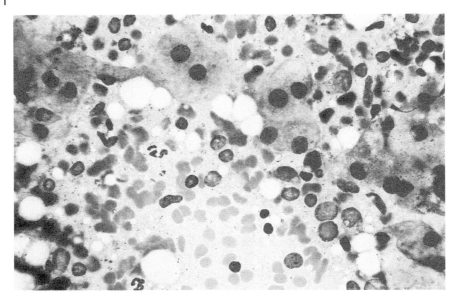

Figure 6.16 Liver, chronic cholangitis, FNCS, dog. Polymorphic lymphocytes and plasma cells are scattered among hepatocytes (MGG, 100×).

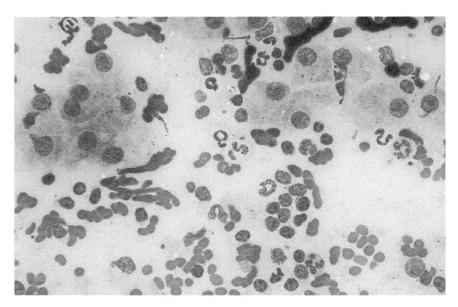

Figure 6.17 Liver, chronic cholangitis, FNCS, dog. Polymorphic lymphocytes together with well-preserved neutrophils (MGG, 100×).

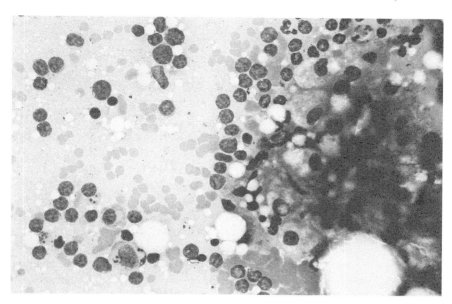

Figure 6.18   Liver, chronic cholangitis, FNCS, dog. Many polymorphic lymphocytes surround hepatocytes with aspecific damage (MGG, 100×).

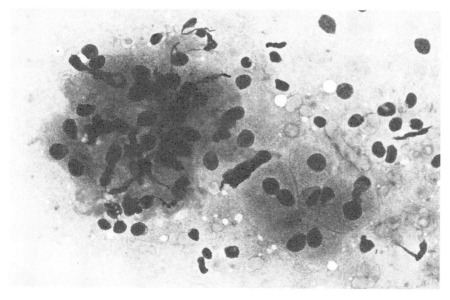

Figure 6.19   Liver, chronic cholangitis, FNCS, dog. Polymorphic lymphocytes surround a group of hepatocytes, crossed by bundles of spindle cells (MGG, 100×).

Table 6.3 Common causes of lymphoplasmacytic inflammation.

Immune-mediated cholangitis
Chronic hepatitis or cholangitis
Viral disease

Together with macrophages, lymphocytes and plasma cells are probably the most common inflammatory categories during subacute and chronic hepatic inflammation (Table 6.3). Some studies on lymphocytic portal infiltration in cat's liver suggest that the causes may be linked to a chronic form of cholangiohepatitis or suppurative cholangiohepatitis, especially when associated with a neutrophilic component. Other studies concerning the periportal infiltration of lymphocytes and plasma cells suggest genetic and immune factors which, after exposure to environmental factors, could predispose some animals to this pathological process [11]. At present, the etiology is unknown but it is believed that genetic and immunological factors may predispose certain animals to produce hepatic lesions after exposure to a variety of environmental factors. Similar to what has been said about neutrophil granulocytes, an attempt to compare them with a peripheral blood leukocyte count would exclude blood contamination and reduce their likely pathological role. The presence of small lymphocytes and plasma cells in a cytological sample is normally a marker of either a subacute or, more likely, a chronic inflammatory process, especially if associated with other inflammatory categories. In some rare cases, fibrosis and apoptosis may be associated conditions (see Chapter 8).

In the course of feline lymphocytic cholangitis (a chronic disease with unknown etiology, probably immunomediated), a high number of (small) lymphocytes may be detected, sometimes with aggregates of epithelial elements of biliary origin (Figure 6.20). The lymphocytes can be found along with plasma cells and sometimes other inflammatory cells close to the hepatocyte aggregates, a circumstance where extracytoplasmic cholestasis can be found in the form of bile casts. The cytological report should include a description of the prevalent lymphocytic and plasma cell inflammation in order to encourage in-depth histopathological studies and allow differential diagnoses, including lymphocytic cholangitis and different forms of chronic hepatitis.

Last but not least, when the lymphocytes are abundant and monomorphic (Figure 6.21), one of the possible differential diagnoses may be primary or metastatic small cell lymphoma. In unclear cases, analysis of the morphological features is insufficient to produce a definitive diagnosis; however, it should be remembered that the cytological sample could represent excellent diagnostic material for biological-molecular evaluations (PCR for antigen receptor

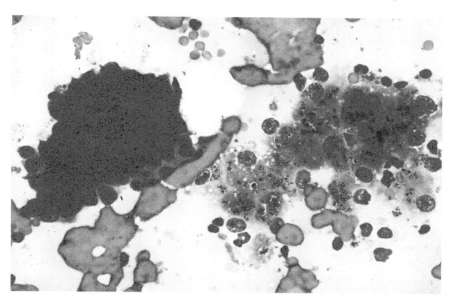

Figure 6.20 Liver, chronic lympocytic cholangitis, FNCS, cat. A large aggregate of biliary cells, with hyperplastic appearance, together with almost normal hepatocytes and some small lymphocytes (MGG, 100×).

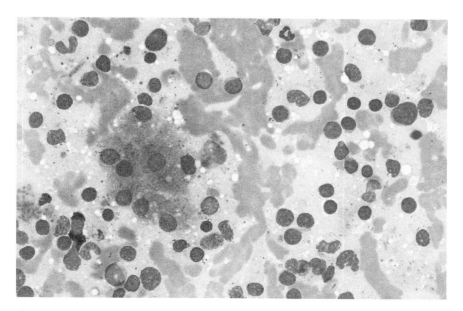

Figure 6.21 Liver, chronic lympocytic cholangitis, FNCS, cat. When a very high number of small lymphocytes is present, a differential diagnosis between a severe form of lymphocytic inflammation and a small cell lymphoma must be determined (MGG, 100×).

rearrangements – PARR method), which would allow investigation of the clonality of the suspected lymphoid population.

6.4 Presence of Macrophages

Cytomorphology: exfoliation of round cells with abundant, irregularly round cytoplasm, filled with achromatic or stained globular material, sometimes in cytophagocytosis (phagocytosis of red blood cell or leukocytes), containing a round, ovoid, cleaved or irregularly shaped nucleus with clumped chromatin (Figure 6.22). Macrophages are scattered on the background, near hepatocyte sheets, frequently associated with other inflammatory cells (Figure 6.23); macrophages may clump in epithelioid aggregates, sometimes together with neutrophils (Figure 6.24), lymphocytes or plasma cells; on the base of the cytoplasmic content, lipogranulomata (cytoplasm filled with achromatic, sharply demarcated lipid globules – Figure 6.25) and pigment granulomata (cytoplasm filled with lipid globules and granules of bluish material – Figure 6.26) may be recognized; siderophages are characterized by cytoplasm filled with gold to brown granular material (Figure 6.27); macrophages may associate with variable degrees of hepatocellular damage (Figure 6.28), fibrosis or cholestasis (Figure 6.29).

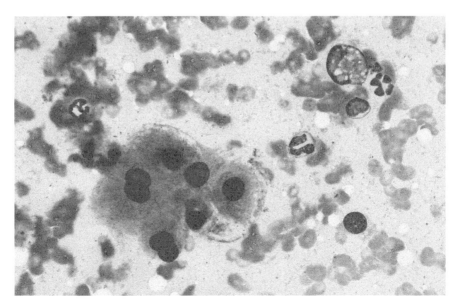

Figure 6.22 Liver, aspecific hepatitis, FNCS, dog. A large macrophage, together with some neutrophils and small lymphocytes. Notice erythrophagocytosis and cytoplasm filled with small globules (MGG, 100×).

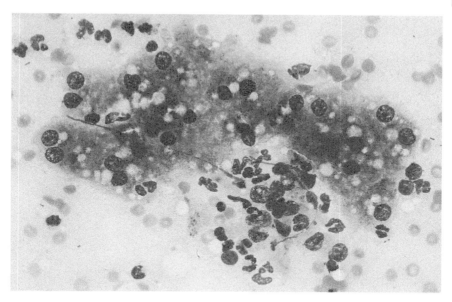

Figure 6.23   Liver, acute mixed hepatitis, unknown causes, FNCS, dog. Macrophages and neutrophils, scattered on the background or aggregated around a cluster of hepatocytes (MGG, 100×).

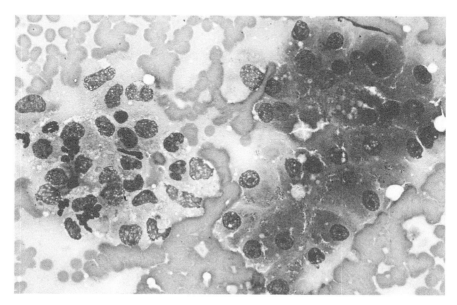

Figure 6.24   Liver, chronic hepatitis, FNCS, dog. An epithelioid aggregate of macrophages (MGG, 100×).

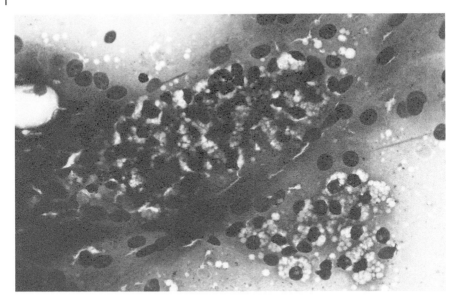

Figure 6.25 Liver, chronic hepatitis, FNCS, dog. Lipogranulomata clustered around a group of hepatocytes (MGG, 100×).

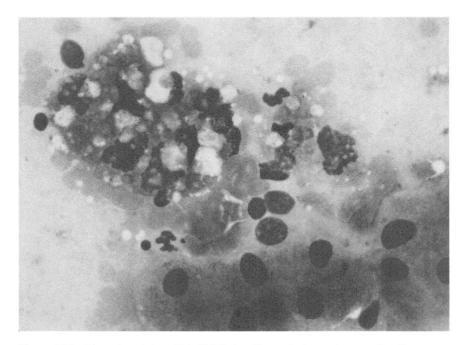

Figure 6.26 Liver, chronic hepatitis, FNCS, dog. Pigmented granuloma; notice the presence of an epithelioid aggregate of enlarged macrophages, with cytoplasm filled with small achromatic globules and bluish pigment (MGG, 100×).

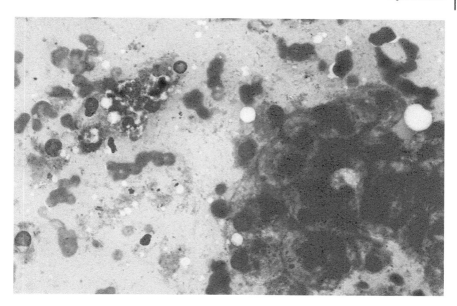

Figure 6.27 Liver, immune-mediated hemolytic anemia, FNCS, dog. An aggregate of siderophages that phagocytized golden to brown material, as a consequence of erythrophagocytosis (MGG, 100×).

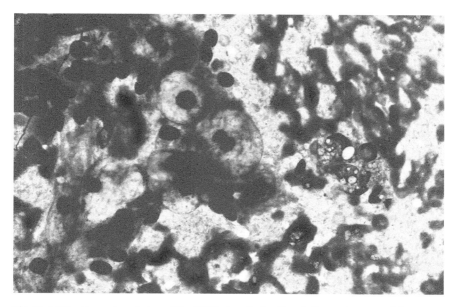

Figure 6.28 Liver, chronic hepatitis, FNCS, dog. As in other inflammatory conditions, macrophages can exfoliate together with hepatocytes that show morphological changes of reversible and aspecific changes (MGG, 100×).

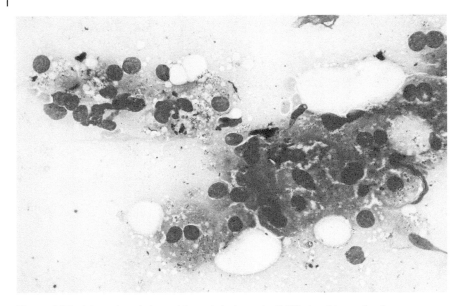

Figure 6.29 Liver, chronic hepatitis and cholestasis, FNCS, dog. Macrophagic cholephagocytosis. Notice bile casts among the hepatocytes (MGG, 100×).

As previously described, Kupffer cells (hepatic resident cells of histiocytic origin) may resemble activated macrophages during inflammatory processes located elsewhere in the body. The activated Kupffer cells are identical to the macrophages that can be detected in other anatomical regions. Single activated macrophages (possibly associated with other inflammatory cells) can be detected in a variety of forms of liver disease (Table 6.4) and their presence is generally nonspecific. Macrophages normally accumulate in the liver, alone or in small groups, as a consequence of damage to the hepatocytes (induced by single cell or focal necrosis, with several potential causes), which is generally nonspecific unless evaluated along with clinical, historical, laboratory data, and ultrasound investigations. The main causes described are toxic, viral, chronic inflammation with fibrosis and neoplastic events [12]. Based on the superior ability of cytology (compared to

Table 6.4 Common causes of macrophagic inflammation.

Fungal diseases
Protozoal diseases
Chronic hepatitis
Unknown causes (most common)

histology) to identify etiological agents, highlighting the activity of phagocytosis by macrophages is relatively easy, especially in the presence of protozoan or fungal origin.

Macrophages can be organized into groups that are variably cohesive, epithelioid in appearance, localized among the aggregates of hepatocytes, or sometimes associated with lymphocytes or neutrophilic granulocytes. This differs from neutrophilic inflammation in that macrophages generally do not infiltrate sheets of hepatocytes. Aggregates of macrophages must be identified and, above all, distinguished from any epithelial aggregates of hepatocellular or biliary origin or even from metastatic epithelium. The recognition criteria are mostly the appearance of the cytoplasm: indistinct, variably expanded, sometimes occupied by achromatic or colored cells and by the polymorphic, predominantly eccentric nucleus profile.

According to published data, granulomatous hepatitis has been reported in association with *Bartonella* spp. [13], *Histoplasma* spp. [14], *Leishmania* spp. [15], and *Mycobacteria* spp. [16]. Recently, *Leptospira* spp. was associated with pyogranulomatous hepatitis without clinical involvement of renal involvement [17]. In my experience, detection of etiological agents that cause granulomatous inflammation, with the exception of *Leishmania* spp., is very rare. Moreover, an infectious cause of granulomatous hepatitis was not identified within liver tissue from 25 dogs using differential staining techniques, fluorescent *in situ* hybridization (FISH) and PCR; in the same study, six out of 25 (24%) dogs were diagnosed with concurrent systemic or localized bacterial infections [18]. Consequently, a diagnosis of granulomatous hepatitis is often accurate but no clear identification of the etiological cause is possible.

Macrophages with cytoplasm filled with ceroid-laden and hemosiderin-laden, foamy, achromatic globules may sometimes form into small epitheloid aggregates defined as "lipogranulomas," together with lymphocytes and plasma cells (Figure 6.30). This is a marker of focal or multifocal damage to the parenchyma (generally nonspecific), where they accumulate and retain the debris that results from focal events of hepatocyte necrosis [19].

From a cytological point of view, it is difficult to distinguish lipogranulomas from the so-called "pigment granulomas": these are epithelial aggregates of macrophages that have engulfed both ceroid and basophilic or brown iron pigment, hemosiderin (Figure 6.31), sometimes together with lymphocytes and plasma cells. Their significance is unknown and they are considered to be a marker of age-related damage.

In the presence of hepatic amyloidosis, the cytoplasm of macrophages may be filled with pink to purple, amorphous to fibrillar material, interpreted to be amyloid since it resembles the material present on the background of the smear; occasional macrophages appeared epithelioid, and contained erythrocytes within the cytoplasm [20].

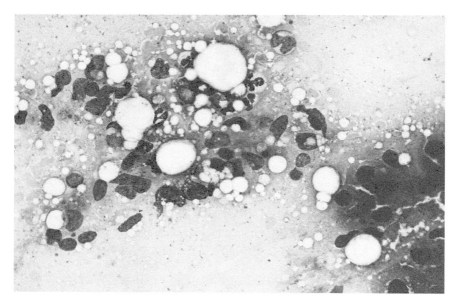

Figure 6.30 Liver, aspecific inflammation, FNCS, dog. A lipogranuloma, where macrophages with enlarged, foamy, fat-containing cytoplasm, exfoliate together with small lymphocytes (MGG, 100×).

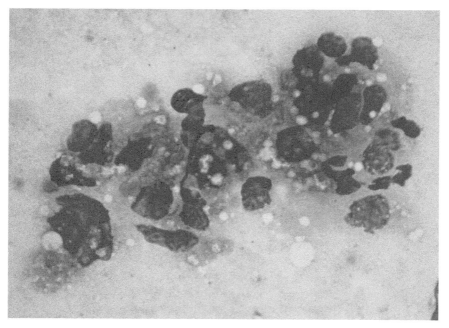

Figure 6.31 Liver, aspecific inflammation, FNCS, dog. A pigment granuloma, containing macrophages with enlarged cytoplasm, filled with round, fatty globules and gray to bluish granules of pigment (MGG, 100×).

6.5 Presence of Mast Cells

Cytomorphology: resident mast cells show small, round cytoplasm filled with coarse metachromatic granules and a round central nucleus with dense chromatin, mostly embedded among hepatocytes (Figure 6.32), sometimes scattered in the background; a very low number of mast cells may be associated with mixed inflammation (Figure 6.33). Association with fibrosis is possible (Figure 6.34).

Mast cells normally live in the hepatic parenchyma and, at least in dogs, tend to be predominantly centrilobular and in very low numbers [21]. The morphological features of hepatic mast cells differ from those of normal mucocutaneous mast cells: they are smaller, with less cytoplasm, which is filled with coarse metachromatic granules and a small round, central nucleus [21]. In cytology and histology, the best way to recognize mast cells is to apply special stains such as toluidine blue, as they accentuate the magenta color of the cytoplasm.

Although sometimes present, scattered on the background, together with mixed inflammation, there is no hepatic inflammatory condition where this cell type is linked to a specific cause. The most common pathological process associated with an increase in the number of mast cells is liver fibrosis (Table 6.5), probably as a consequence of the role of this cell in chronic damage and fibrosis [22, 23].

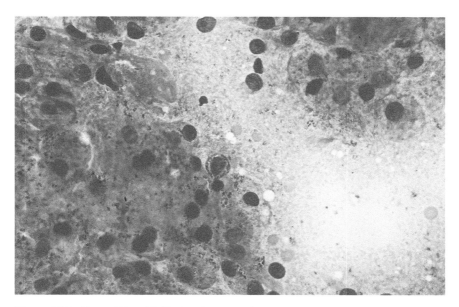

Figure 6.32 Normal liver, FNCS, dog. A normal liver mast cell among the hepatocytes (MGG, 100×).

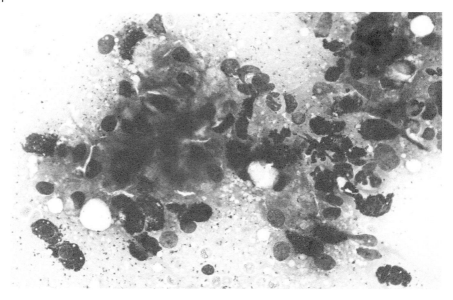

Figure 6.33 Liver, reactive aspecific hepatitis, FNCS, dog. Mast cells exfoliate together with other inflammatory cells (MGG, 100×).

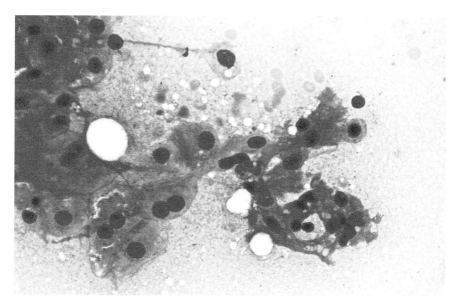

Figure 6.34 Liver, fibrosis, FNCS, dog. A single mast cell close to a bundle of spindle cells (MGG, 100×).

Table 6.5 Common causes of increased number of mast cells.

Liver fibrosis

Mast cell metastasis

The presence of mast cells, especially when they are numerous and found in clusters between the hepatocytes, should be attributed possibly to primary or metastatic mast cell tumors, as described in Chapter 12.

6.6 Key Points

- Inflammation is the most difficult pathological process to be assessed by cytological examination; be careful when trying to diagnose an inflammatory hepatopathy without histological examination.
- The most important condition to be differentiated from a true inflammation is the presence of leukocytes from blood contamination.
- Neutrophilic granulocytes assume great diagnostic power in recognition of a septic hepatitis when degenerated or in phagocytosis of bacteria.
- The very rare cases of eosinophilic inflammation are caused by hypersensitivity conditions from parasitic migration or by adverse reaction to drugs.
- Lymphocytic inflammation is generally aspecific. In cats, a high number of polymorphic lymphocytes should be associated with a diagnosis of lymphocytic cholangitis.
- Macrophagic inflammation is generally aspecific. In most cases a primary cause is not recognizable.

References

1 Wang, K.Y., Panciera, D.L., Al-Rukibat, R.K. et al. (2004). Accuracy of ultrasound-guided fine-needle aspiration of the liver and cytologic findings in dogs and cats: 97 cases (1990–2000). *J. Am. Vet. Med. Assoc.* 224: 75–78.
2 Weiss, D.J., Blauvelt, M., and Aird, B. (2001). Cytologic evaluation of inflammation in canine liver aspirates. *Vet. Clin. Pathol.* 30: 193–196.
3 Van den Ingh, T.S.G.A.M., van Winkle, T., Cullen, J.M. et al. (2006). Morphological classification of parenchymal disorders of the canine and feline liver – hepatocellular death, hepatitis and cirrhosis. In: *Standard for Clinical and Histological Diagnosis of Canine and Feline Liver Disease* (ed. WSAVA Liver Standardization Group), 90–91. St Louis, MO: Saunders.

4 Gardner, R.H., Castillo, D., Constantino-Casas, F., and Williams, T.L. (2022). Can the neutrophil count from hepatic fine-needle aspirate cytology be used to diagnose hepatitis in dogs? A pilot study. *Vet. Clin. Pathol.* 51: 237–243.

5 Masserdotti, C. (2020). The cytologic features of biliary diseases: a retrospective study. *Vet. Clin. Pathol.* 49 (3): 440–450.

6 Arndt, T.P. and Shelly, S.M. (2014). *The Liver. Diagnostic Cytology of the Dog and Cat*, 4e, 358–359. St Louis, MO: Elsevier Mosby.

7 Meyer, D.K. (2016). The liver. In: *Canine and Feline Cytology – A Color Atlas and Interpretation Guide*, 3e (ed. R. Raskin and D. Meyer), 259–283. St Louis, MO: Elsevier.

8 Giordano, A., Paltrinieri, S., Bertazzolo, W. et al. (2005). Sensitivity of Tru-cut and fine needle aspiration biopsies of liver and kidney for diagnosis of feline infectious peritonitis. *Vet. Clin. Pathol.* 34 (4): 368–374.

9 Irvine, K.L., Walker, J.M., and Friedrichs, K.R. (2016). Sarcocystid organisms found in bile from a dog with acute hepatitis: a case report and review of intestinal and hepatobiliary Sarcocystidae infections in dogs and cats. *Vet. Clin. Pathol.* 45 (1): 57–65.

10 Allison, R., Williams, P., Lansdowne, J. et al. (2006). Fatal hepatic sarcocystosis in a puppy with eosinophilia and eosinophilic peritoneal effusion. *Vet. Clin. Pathol.* 35 (3): 353–357.

11 Lucke, V.M. and Davies, J.D. (1984). Progressive lymphocytic cholangitis in the cat. *J. Small Anim. Pract.* 25: 249–260.

12 Elchaninov, A.V., Fatkhudinov, T.K., Vishnyakova, P.A. et al. (2019). Phenotypical and functional polymorphism of liver resident macrophages. *Cells* 8 (9): 1032.

13 Gillespie, T.N., Thornburn, D., Oien, K.A. et al. (2003). Detection of Bartonella henselae and Bartonella clarridgeiae DNA in hepatic specimens from two dogs with hepatic disease. *J. Am. Vet. Med. Assoc.* 222 (35): 47–51.

14 Brömel, C. and Sykes, J.E. (2005). Histoplasmosis in dogs and cats. *Clin. Tech. Small Anim. Pract.* 20 (4): 227–232.

15 Rallis, T., Day, M.J., Saridomichelakis, M.N. et al. (2005). Chronic hepatitis associated with canine leishmaniosis (Leishmania infantum): a clinicopathological study of 26 cases. *J. Comp. Pathol.* 132 (2–3): 145–152.

16 Eggers, J.S., Parker, G.A., Braaf, H.A., and Mense, M.G. (1997). Disseminated Mycobacterium avium infection in three miniature schnauzer litter mates. *J. Vet. Diagn. Invest.* 9: 424–427.

17 McCallum, K.E., Constantino-Casas, F., Cullen, J.M. et al. (2019). Hepatic leptospiral infections in dogs without obvious renal involvement. *J. Vet. Intern. Med.* 33 (1): 141–150.

18 Hutchins, R.G., Breitschwerdt, E.B., Cullen, J.M. et al. (2012). Limited yield of diagnoses of intrahepatic infectious causes of canine granulomatous hepatitis from archival liver tissue. *J. Vet. Diagn. Invest.* 24 (5): 888–894.

19 Van Winkle, T., Cullen, J.M., van den Ingh, T.S.G.A.M. et al. (2006). Morphological classification of parenchymal disorders of the canine and feline liver – hepatic abcesses and granulomas, hepatic metabolic storage disorders and miscellaneous conditions. In: *Standard for Clinical and Histological Diagnosis of Canine and Feline Liver Disease* (ed. WSAVA Liver Standardization Group), 103–116. St Louis, MO: Saunders.

20 Neo-Suzuki, S., Mineshige, T., Kamiie, J. et al. (2017). Hepatic AA amyloidosis in a cat: cytologic and histologic identification of AA amyloid in macrophages. *Vet. Clin. Pathol.* 46 (2): 331–336.

21 Yamamoto, K. (2000). Electron microscopy of mast cells in the venous wall of canine liver. *J. Vet. Med. Sci.* 62 (11): 1183–1188.

22 Masserdotti, C. (2013). Proportion of mast cells in normal canine hepatic cytologic specimens: comparison of 2 staining methods. *Vet. Clin. Pathol.* 42 (4): 522–525.

23 Masserdotti, C. and Bertazzolo, W. (2016). Cytologic features of hepatic fibrosis in dogs: a retrospective study on 22 cases. *Vet. Clin. Pathol.* 45 (2): 361–367.

7

Nuclear Inclusions

Rarely does the nucleus of the hepatocyte undergo morphological alterations related to ongoing pathological process, not even during serious degenerative alterations, such as pyknosis and karyorrhexis, inflammatory processes or neoplastic transformations. In this chapter, I analyze the most frequent irregularities of the nucleus, in particular nuclear inclusions and nuclear pseudo-inclusions – structures of variable appearance located within the nucleus of the hepatocyte. True nuclear inclusions must be differentiated from a prominent nucleolus and from chromatin clumps.

7.1 "Brick" Inclusions

Cytomorphology: rectangular crystal-like appearance, measuring between 10 and 15 μm (size may vary considerably) that can deform the nuclear profile (Figure 7.1). They can be found in the nuclei of completely normal hepatocytes.

These inclusions are relatively frequent and affect individual sporadic hepatocytes. Despite being frequently detected, they should be considered incidental findings with no currently known clinical implications. First described in 1902 by Tadeusz Browicz, these structures have been discussed [1] and subsequently subjected to immunohistochemical investigation, which suggested they may be of proteinaceous nature [2], thus excluding mineral or lipid derivation, as well as possible connections with DNA, RNA, cholesterol, glycogen, mucin, mucopolysaccharides, polysaccharides, glycoproteins, glycolipids, and hemoglobin [3]. Their proteinaceous nature has been hypothetically associated with three different events: the accumulation of proteins in crystallized form (the accumulation process being faster than the expulsion process, through the nuclear membrane), the synthesis and accumulation of proteins in crystalline form or an excess of

Canine and Feline Liver Cytology, First Edition. Carlo Masserdotti.
© 2024 John Wiley & Sons, Inc. Published 2024 by John Wiley & Sons, Inc.

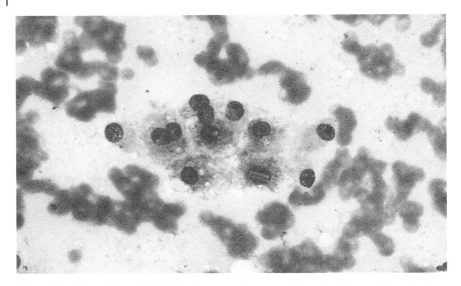

Figure 7.1 Normal liver, FNCS, dog. Presence of rectangular, refractile crystals called "brick inclusion" inside the nucleus of a hepatocyte (MGG, 100×).

proteins caused by pathological processes. To date, however, none of these possibilities has been demonstrated.

Crystalline inclusions are typical of dogs and have not been observed in other species. Although they have never been demonstrated, it is hypothesized that they may be the result of a hereditary defect or the consequence of permanent protein damage caused by viral infections or even crystallization of proteins of viral origin [4].

7.2 Glycogen Pseudo-inclusions

Cytomorphology: small achromatic or weakly eosinophilic bodies located in the nucleus with a roundish profile (Figure 7.2). They may be found within the nuclei of hepatocytes affected by cytoplasmic glycogen accumulation (Figure 7.3), but may also be present in cells of normal appearance. In the nucleus, they are caused by the invagination of cytoplasmic material.

In cytology, these are extremely rare nuclear irregularities and some texts associate them with diabetes mellitus or neoplastic transformation. I do not have any personal experience concerning their causes.

Recent studies have identified the presence of glycogen pseudo-inclusions within the nucleus of gastric epithelial cells, which was considered incidental [5].

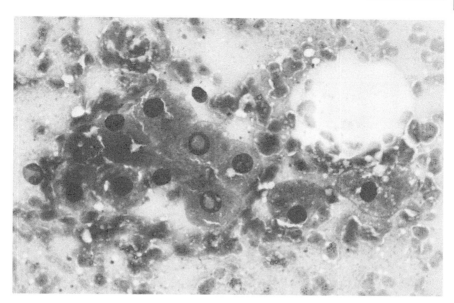

Figure 7.2   Liver, reversible aspecific injury, FNCS, dog. Two large, pale, round inclusions, inside the nucleus of the central hepatocytes (MGG, 100×).

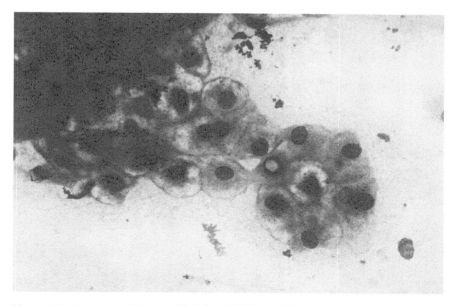

Figure 7.3   Liver, reversible aspecific injury, FNCS, dog. A large, pale, roundish nuclear inclusion; notice the presence of achromatic material inside the cytoplasm (MGG, 100×).

7.3 Lead Inclusions

This type of intranuclear inclusion may be observed occasionally in dogs with lead intoxication. The inclusions, mostly present in the epithelial cells of proximal renal tubules and osteoblasts, can be rarely observed in liver tissue; in some cases the Ziehl–Neelsen stain can help in recognition of acid-fast inclusions [6]. I have never experienced this observation in my practice.

7.4 Viral Inclusions

Cytomorphology: dense, homogeneous, irregularly rounded eosinophilic or basophilic bodies of variable size; visibly different from the nucleolus, which is generally small or inconsistent and always basophilic (Figure 7.4). They may be associated with nonspecific hepatocellular damage and inflammatory conditions.

Adenoviruses are one cause of the most easily identified intranuclear inclusions. Canine adenoviruses (CAdVs) include type 1 (CAdV-1, virulent strain) and type 2

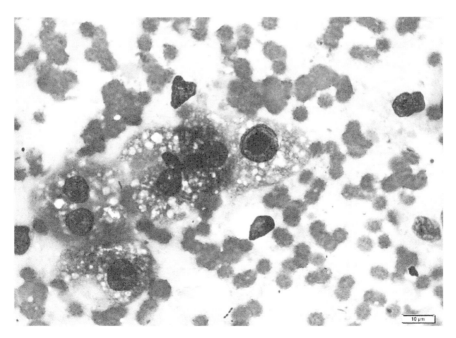

Figure 7.4 Liver, adenovirus hepatitis, FNCS, dog. A large eosinophilic inclusion in the nucleus of the hepatocyte to the right (MGG, 100×). *Source:* Courtesy of Dr Marian Taulescu.

(CAdV-2, attenuated strain), which induce canine hepatitis and tracheobronchitis respectively. CAdV-1 and CAdV-2 have the same genome structure, diameter, morphological features, and cytopathic features but have different genome sequence, coding proteins, viral activity, and hemagglutination patterns. Sequence alignment, PCR, and real-time-PCR assay are useful methods to distinguish the two serotypes [7]; immunohistochemistry staining for CAdV-1 and CAdV-2 is also useful [8].

Infectious canine hepatitis has a worldwide distribution and is spread by direct or indirect contact. Clinical signs include fever, anorexia, vomiting, diarrhea, and abdominal pain, although ocular (unilateral or bilateral opacity of the cornea, caused by corneal edema, the so-called "blue eye") and neurological signs have been described [8]. In an affected puppy, histopathology performed on the liver revealed the presence of diffusely and mildly "vacuolated" hepatocytes; rare individual cell necrosis was observed and hepatocyte nuclei also frequently contained large acidophilic inclusion bodies with a blue tint [9]. Herpesviruses, paramyxoviruses, and parvoviruses also cause multisystemic diseases involving the liver of dog [10–12] and cat [13].

7.5 Key Points

- The most frequent nuclear inclusions observed are the so-called "brick" and glycogen pseudo-inclusions.
- Other inclusions are very rarely observed in daily practice. When present, care must be taken to differentiate true inclusions from a prominent nucleolus or chromatin clumps.

References

1 Browicz, T. (1902). Meine Ansichten uber den Bau der Lebenzelle. *Virchow Arch. Pathol. Anat.* 168: 1–22.
2 Thompson, S.W. II, Wiegand, R.G., Thomassen, R.W. et al. (1959). The protein nature of acidophilic crystalline intranuclear inclusions in the liver and kidney of dogs. *Am. J. Pathol.* 35: 1105–1115.
3 Thompson, S.W., Cook, J.E., and Hoey, H. (1959). Histochemical studies of acidophilic crystalline intranuclear inclusions in the liver and kidney of dogs. *Am. J. Pathol.* 35: 607–623.
4 Richter, W.R., Stein, R.J., Rdzok, E.J. et al. (1965). Ultrastructural studies of intranuclear crystalline inclusions in the liver of the dog. *Am. J. Pathol.* 47 (4): 587–599.

5 Silvestri, S., Lepri, E., Dall'Aglio, C. et al. (2017). Nuclear glycogen inclusions in canine parietal cells. *Vet. Pathol.* 54 (3): 520–526.

6 Hamir, A.N., Sullivan, N.D., and Handson, P.D. (1983). Acid fast inclusions in tissues of dogs dosed with lead. *J. Comp. Pathol.* 93 (2): 307–317.

7 Zhu, Y., Jinfeng, X., Lian, S. et al. (2022). Difference analysis between canine adenovirus types 1 and 2. *Front. Cell. Infect. Microbiol.* 11 (12): 854–876.

8 Hornsey, S.J., Philibert, H., Godson, D.L., and Snead, E.C.R. (2019). Canine adenovirus type 1 causing neurological signs in a 5-week-old puppy. *BMC Vet. Res.* 15 (1): 418.

9 Cullen, J.M. and Stalker, M.J. (2016). Liver and biliary system. In: *Jubb, Kennedy and Palmer's Pathology of Domestic Animals*, VIe (ed. M.G. Maxie), 310–311. St Louis, MO: Elsevier.

10 Barbie, J., Gadsden, B.J., Maes, R.K. et al. (2012). Fatal Canid herpesvirus 1 infection in an adult dog. *J. Vet. Diagn. Invest.* 24 (3): 604–607.

11 Kobayashi, Y., Ochiai, K., and Itakura, C. (1993). Dual infection with canine distemper virus and infectious canine hepatitis virus (canine adenovirus type 1) in a dog. *J. Vet. Med. Sci.* 55 (4): 699–701.

12 Nho, W.G., Sur, J.H., Doster, A.R., and Kim, S.B. (1997). Detection of canine parvovirus in naturally infected dogs with enteritis and myocarditis by in situ hybridization. *J. Vet. Diagn. Invest.* 9 (3): 255–260.

13 Bestetti, G. and Zwahlen, R. (1985). Generalized parvovirus infection with inclusion-body myocarditis in two kittens. *J. Comp. Pathol.* 95 (3): 393–397.

8

Cytological Features of Liver Fibrosis

The undiscussed predominance of histopathological evaluations makes hepatic fibrosis a thorny topic for cytology. Despite being insufficient for the formulation of specific diagnoses, cytology can provide useful information about the presence of hepatic fibrosis and represent the starting point for a definitive diagnosis of a chronic, severe, generally irreversible pathological process by histological examination.

Hepatic fibrosis is the result of chronic inflammation combined with hepatocellular necrosis and apoptosis. Liver fibrosis is not a specific disease but rather the result of conditions that determine the expansion of stromal support of the portal or centro-lobular tracts, the formation of fibrous branches that interconnect adjacent portal spaces (porto-portal fibrosis) or the portal spaces with centro-lobular spaces (porto-central fibrosis). Fibrosis may be extensive and sometimes the direction of its branches is not easily distinguished without the use of special stains, such as golden trichromic. In severe cases, the hepatocytes may even be arranged in aggregates or small groups surrounded by connective bundles, as in end-stage fibrosis (or cirrhosis), or isolated, as in lobular dissecting hepatitis.

The conditions that lead to hepatic fibrosis include all pathological processes responsible for chronic and possibly irreversible damage: infectious conditions, toxins, adverse reactions to drugs, chronic cholangiopathies, immune-mediated injury, and accumulation of copper, among others. Fibrosis is the morphological expression of chronic injury. Additional clinical and historical data, as well as laboratory, ultrasonographic and histopathological investigations, are often necessary for a final diagnosis.

The role of cytology is to make the most of the data derived from the analysis of cell morphology and to provide as many indications about the *presence* of fibrosis in the hepatic parenchyma as possible. The aim is to refrain from attempting causal diagnosis, delegating the recognition of any primary causes, direction and extension of the event to histology, if possible. We could say that, similarly to

Canine and Feline Liver Cytology, First Edition. Carlo Masserdotti.
© 2024 John Wiley & Sons, Inc. Published 2024 by John Wiley & Sons, Inc.

cholestasis or nonspecific hepatocellular damage, fibrosis is just a peculiar cyto-morphological feature; however, in order to correctly hypothesize primary causes and recognize associated changes, such as necroinflammatory activity, distribution of fibrotic branches or chronic cholangitis, histological examination is mandatory.

8.1 Cytological Features of Liver Fibrosis

Cytomorphology: presence of spindle cells arranged in linear or branched bundles, crossing the hepatocyte aggregates or interconnecting groups of hepatocytes (Figure 8.1); spindle cells show eosinophilic cytoplasm, which is sometimes filled with brown to black microgranules (Figure 8.2), and contains ovoid nuclei with finely granular or compact chromatin (Figure 8.3); spindle cells are embedded in pink, fibrillary, eosinophilic strands (Figure 8.4); single mast cells with small amount of irregularly granular cytoplasm and round nucleus are sometimes located near the bundles of spindle cells (Figure 8.5); the hepatocytes are frequently affected by reversible nonspecific damage (Figures 8.6 and 8.7); possible focal necrotic phenomena or apoptotic hepatocytes (Figure 8.8); cholestasis is possible, although rare (Figure 8.9); the presence of inflammatory cells is an inconstant finding (Figure 8.10).

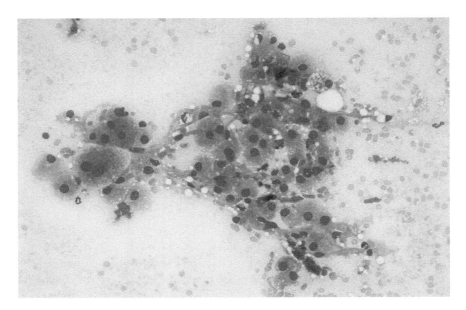

Figure 8.1 Liver, chronic hepatitis, FNCS, dog. A cluster of hepatocytes crossed by branched bundles of spindle cells and pink fibrillary material (MGG, 40×).

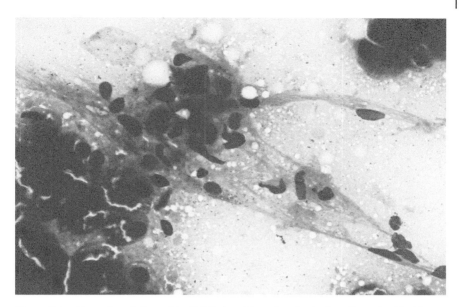

Figure 8.2 Liver, chronic hepatitis, FNCS, dog. A bundle of spindle cells embedded in pink fibrillary material; notice the presence of small granules inside the cytoplasm of a spindle cell at the bottom (MGG, 100×).

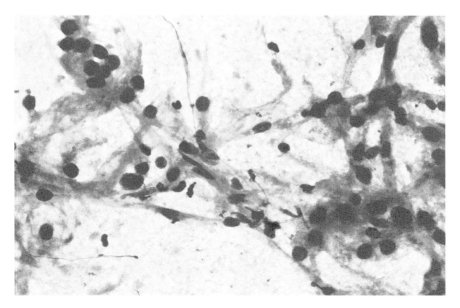

Figure 8.3 Liver, chronic hepatitis, FNCS, dog. A web of spindle cells, with eosinophilic cytoplasm and small, round to ovoid nucleus, with compact chromatin (MGG, 100×).

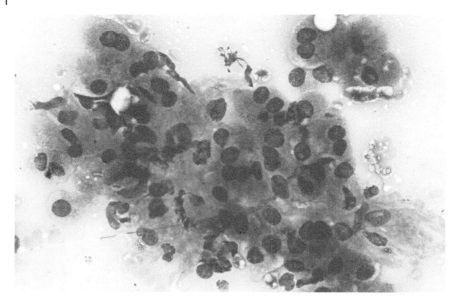

Figure 8.4 Liver, chronic hepatitis, FNCS, dog. Fibrillary material, probably represented by stroma, may exfoliate in variable amounts (MGG, 100×).

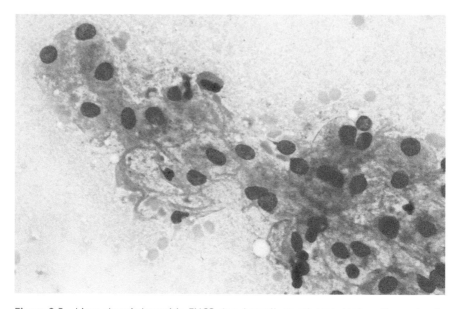

Figure 8.5 Liver, chronic hepatitis, FNCS, dog. A small, round, granular hepatic mast cell, on the top, exfoliates close to the spindle cells that interconnect two groups of hepatocytes (MGG, 100×).

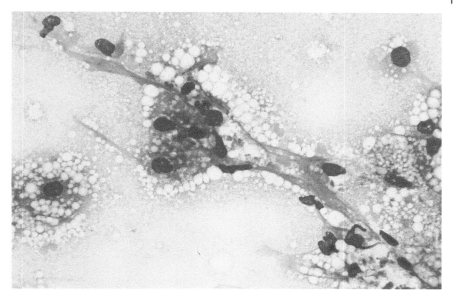

Figure 8.6 Liver, chronic hepatitis, FNCS, dog. A bundle of spindle cells are close to steatotic hepatocytes; lipid material is also scattered on the background (MGG, 100×).

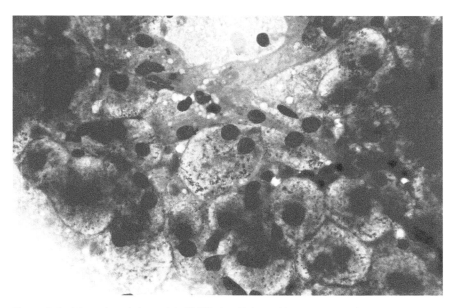

Figure 8.7 Liver, chronic hepatitis, FNCS, dog. Enlarged hepatocytes, with reversible injury, crossed by spindle cells (MGG, 100×).

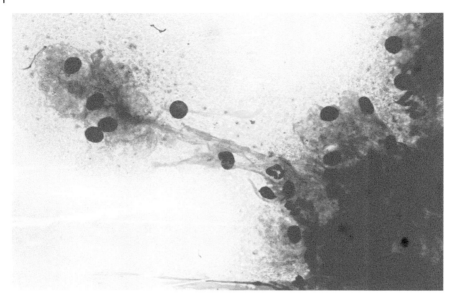

Figure 8.8 Liver, chronic hepatitis, FNCS, dog. An apoptotic hepatocyte, to the left of the right cluster, with deep eosinophilic cytoplasm and shrunken nucleus, close to the spindle cells (MGG, 100×).

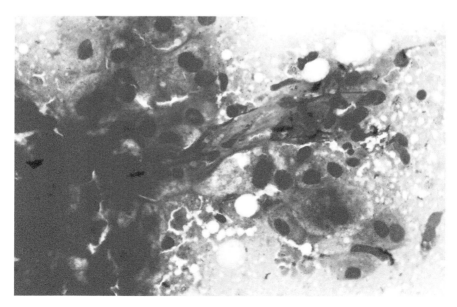

Figure 8.9 Liver, chronic hepatitis, FNCS, dog. Casts of biliary material may accumulate close to hepatocytes and spindle cells (MGG, 100×).

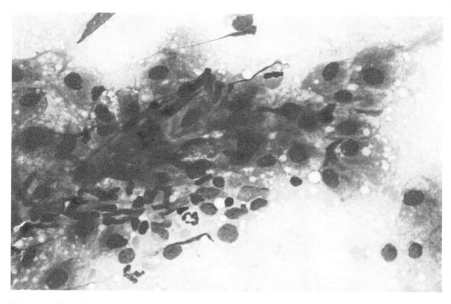

Figure 8.10   Liver, chronic hepatitis, FNCS, dog. The presence of inflammatory cells close to hepatocytes and spindle cells can be seen (MGG, 100×).

Liver fibrosis is an increase in the components of fibrillar extracellular matrix, such as collagen, structural glycoproteins. and proteoglycans, with the initial deposition in the subendothelial space of Disse, leading to the formation of a diffusion barrier between hepatocytes and sinusoid structures [1]. Furthermore, it includes a reparative cicatricial process to the parenchyma, resulting from a variety of inflammatory stimuli such as persistent infections, autoimmune reactions and tissue damage induced by toxic or pharmacological molecules [2] (Figure 8.11).

Specific causes of hepatic fibrosis in the dog [3] are briefly described in Table 8.1. The onset and progression mechanisms normally include the activation of hepatic stellate cells (also called Ito cells) [4, 5] and their transdifferentiation into myofibroblasts [6]. Myofibroblasts may originate from portal [7] or central [8] mesenchymal cells too. The activation of hepatic stellate cells is a consequence of the paracrine activity triggered by activation of cytokines, which are released by necrotic and probably apoptotic hepatocytes [9], as well as by the action of cytokines released by leukocytes, thrombocytes, and Kupffer cells. This transformation gives hepatic stellate cells their spindle appearance and contractile potential, due to cytoplasmic increase of smooth muscle actin and ability to secrete a wide range of extracellular matrix components, as well as numerous pro- and antiinflammatory cytokines and growth factors. In addition, there is well-established evidence that the transformation of stellate hepatic cells into myofibroblasts is accompanied by epithelial–mesenchymal transition (EMT)

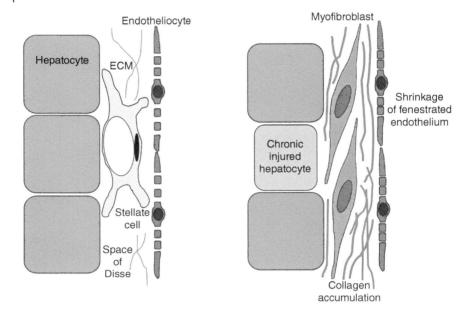

Figure 8.11 In normal liver, stellate (Ito) cells are indicated by cytoplasmic globules, where vitamin A is stored (left). After chronic hepatocyte damage, stellate cells transform into myofibroblasts and produce extracellular matrix components, leading to the formation of fibrosis (right).

Table 8.1 Common causes of hepatic fibrosis in dogs.

Chronic hepatitis
- Caused by copper accumulation (about 30% of dogs)
- No underlying demonstrable causes (about 60% of dogs)

Lobular dissecting hepatitis

Chronic extrahepatic bile duct obstruction

Chronic cholangitis

Right-sided heart failure

Ductal plate abnormalities
- Congenital hepatic fibrosis

Source: Adapted from [3].

phenomena, which lead to the transformation of cholangiocytes and hepatocytes into fibroblasts [1].

Whatever their origin, myofibroblast and other fibrogenic cell types are activated by a large number of mediator-producing inflammatory events, including cytokines (IL-13, IL-21, TGF-beta-1), chemokines (MCP-1), angiogenetic factors (VEGF), growth factors (PDGF), and acute-phase proteins, stimulating the production of collagen [6]. During the initial stages of fibrogenesis, the deposition of extracellular matrix mostly involves the Disse space (the transition area between the endotheliocytes of the liver sinusoids and the surface membrane of the hepatocyte), causing a decrease in fenestrations which alters the metabolic exchanges – often called "sinusoidal capillarization" as the sinusoids resemble vascular capillaries [10]. This cellular activation triggers a complex process that results in the deposition of extracellular matrix and the consequent formation of various microanatomical connective bundles between the hepatocytes: porto-portal extensions (between two adjacent portal spaces); porto-central extensions (between a portal space and the corresponding centro-lobular vessel), or centro-central extensions (between two centro-lobular areas).

The term "cirrhosis," the end-stage of chronic hepatitis, refers to the development of a fibrotic process (Figures 8.12 and 8.13), which results in the conversion of normal liver architecture into irregular regenerative nodules and bridging fibrosis, as well as the development of porto-central vascular anastomoses [11, 12].

An increased number of spindle-shaped cells observed in a cytological sample from canine fibrotic liver derive from these cellular transformations and evolutions. A complete description of the cytological features of liver fibrosis was

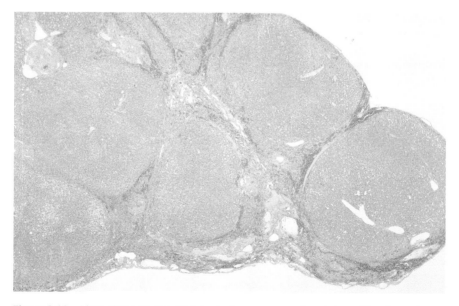

Figure 8.12   Liver, cirrhosis, dog. Histological appearance of end-stage fibrosis; notice the presence of newly formed septa of fibrous tissue (HE, 20×).

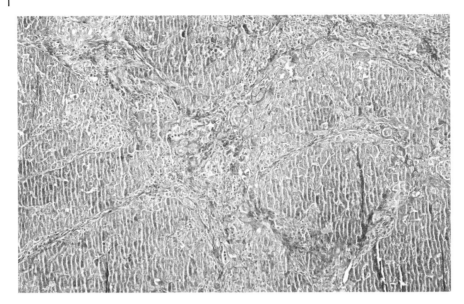

Figure 8.13   Liver, cirrhosis, dog. Fibrous tissue appears green with special stain (Masson-Fontana, 40×).

given by Masserdotti and Bertazzolo [13]. In this paper, a spindle cell/hepatocyte mean ratio of 0.336 was calculated in liver with fibrosis, compared with a mean ratio of 0.012 in nonfibrotic liver [13]. The morphological findings described are insufficient to provide indications about the extent and degree of the fibrotic activation processes, but they may be enough to justify further clinical efforts aimed at investigating the ongoing hepatic disease through additional histopathological diagnostic tools.

The presence of cytoplasmic granules in the cytoplasm of spindle cells may be a marker of an increased presence of enzymes and inflammatory mediators of the myofibroblast, although this hypothesis requires further research and confirmation. In the scientific literature, the presence of an increased number of mast cells in liver fibrosis is attributed to the key role played by these cells both in fibrotic processes and the course of acute inflammatory phenomena [14–16]. In particular, during fibrosis, they promote the growth of fibroblasts and stimulate stellate cells to produce extracellular matrix [17]. The presence of mast cells has been described in cases of canine nonspecific reactive hepatitis, in destructive cholangitis, cirrhosis, and chronic hepatitis [18, 19]; in addition, their important role in the sinusoidal capillarization process is recognized [18]. An increased number of mast cells has been detected in cases of canine liver fibrosis [13]. When evaluating a hepatic cytological sample during cutaneous mast cell tumor staging, it is important to remember this information, as failure to do so may lead to attributing the presence of these cells (especially if considerable) to metastatic reasons and not to fibrosis.

The degenerative changes of the hepatocytes, namely the accumulation of glycogen, water, lipids or lipofuscin, are generally ascribed to hypoxic conditions or to the causes of the ongoing pathological process. Moreover, it is sometimes possible to observe very rare apoptotic hepatocytes in the aggregates near the bundles of spindle cells; this finding is related to the chronic stage of hepatitis, where apoptosis or necrosis is a constant change. When present on slides, recognition of apoptotic cells, represented by shrunken, hyperchromatic cells with collapsed nucleus, may be difficult.

Cholestasis is a uncommon finding in cytological specimens; although easy to identify and represented by the presence of bluish-greenish casts among the hepatocytes, this finding is not frequently observed [13]. This uncommon recognition of cholestasis should be related to the fact that, in many cases, a concomitant reactive proliferation of bile ducts accompanies the fibrosis process, leading to a normal deflux of bile. In dogs affected with chronic hepatitis, bile was not observed histologically in the canaliculi in 16 of 22 dogs [20]; moreover, in the same study, hyperbilirubinemia was present in only seven of the 22 dogs.

The number of inflammatory cells is extremely variable in samples from liver with fibrosis [13]; when present, a mixed population of macrophages, lymphocytes, plasma cells, and neutrophils may be evident. This could be explained by the fact that fibrosis is a consequence of many inflammatory conditions and independent of the action of specific inflammatory cell populations. In fact, the onset of fibrosis is mostly a direct consequence of the duration of the inflammatory activity, and thus the inflammatory cell population may be low in chronic conditions.

8.2   Key Points

- Liver fibrosis is indicated by the presence of spindle cells and bundles of eosinophilic strands among the hepatocytes.
- Near to the bundles of spindle cells, the presence of single mast cells is a frequent finding.
- The presence of inflammatory cells is an inconstant finding.
- The presence of cytological evidence for fibrosis should lead to further investigation, by histopathological examination, in order to stage and grade the degree and extent of the fibrosis and, whenever possible, to individuate primary causes.

References

1 Gressner, O.A., Weiskirchen, R., and Gressner, A.M. (2007). Evolving concepts of liver fibrogenesis provide new diagnostic and therapeutic options. *Comp. Hepatol.* 6: 7.

2 Van den Ingh, T.S.G.A.M., van Winkle, T.V., Cullen, J.M. et al. (2006). Morphological classification of parenchymal disorders of the canine and feline liver. In: *WSAVA Standards for the Clinical and Histological Diagnosis of Canine and Feline Liver Disease* (ed. WSAVA Liver Standardization Group), 85–103. Philadelphia, PA: Saunders Elsevier.

3 Eulenberg, V.M. and Lidbury, J.A. (2018). Hepatic fibrosis in dogs. *J. Vet. Intern. Med.* 32 (1): 26–41.

4 Kmiec, Z. (2001). Cooperation of liver cells in health and disease. *Adv. Anat. Embryol. Cell Biol.* 161: III–XIII, 1–151.

5 Senoo, H. (2004). Structure and function of hepatic stellate cells. *Med. Electron Microsc.* 37: 3–15.

6 Wynn, T. (2008). Cellular and molecular mechanism of fibrosis. *J. Pathol.* 214: 199–210.

7 Lemoinne, S., Cadoret, A., El Mourabit, H. et al. (2013). Origins and functions of liver myofibroblasts. *Biochim. Biophys. Acta* 1832 (7): 948–954.

8 Asahina, K., Zhou, B., Pu, W.T., and Tsukamoto, H. (2011). Septum transversum-derived mesothelium gives rise to hepatic stellate cells and perivascular mesenchymal cells in developing mouse liver. *Hepatology* 53 (3): 983–995.

9 Roth, S., Michel, K., and Gressner, A.M. (1998). Latent transforming growth factor-beta in liver parenchymal cells, its injury-dependent release and paracrine effects on hepatic stellate cells. *Hepatology* 27: 1003–1012.

10 Varin, F. and Huet, P.M. (1985). Hepatic microcirculation in the perfused cirrhotic rat liver. *J. Clin. Invest.* 76: 1904–1912.

11 Anthony, H.D., Ishak, K.G., Nayak, N.C. et al. (1977). The morphology of cirrhosis: definition, nomenclature and classification. *Bull. World Health Organ.* 55: 521–540.

12 Craword, J.M. (2002). Liver cirrhosis. In: *Pathology of the Liver*, 4e (ed. R.N.M. McSween, A.D. Burt, and B.C. Portmann), 575–620. Edinburgh: Churchill Livingstone.

13 Masserdotti, C. and Bertazzolo, W. (2016). Cytologic features of hepatic fibrosis in dogs: a retrospective study on 22 cases. *Vet. Clin. Pathol.* 45 (2): 361–367.

14 Matsunaga, Y., Kawasaki, H., and Terada, T. (1999). Stromal mast cells and nerve fibers in various chronic liver diseases: relevance to hepatic fibrosis. *Am. J. Gastroenterol.* 94: 1923–1932.

15 Grizzi, F., Franceschini, B., Barbieri, B. et al. (2002). Mast cell density: a quantitative index of acute liver inflammation. *Anal. Quant. Cytol. Histol.* 24: 63–69.

16 Farrell, D.J., Hines, J.E., Walls, A.F. et al. (1995). Intrahepatic mast cells in chronic liver diseases. *Hepatology* 22 (4 Pt 1): 1175–1181.

17 Jeong, D.H., Lee, G.P., Jeong, W.I. et al. (2005). Alterations of mast cells and TGF-beta1 on the silymarin treatment for CCl (4)-induced hepatic fibrosis. *World J. Gastroenterol.* 11: 1141–1148.

18 Stockhaus, C., van den Ingh, T., Rothuizen, J., and Teske, E. (2004). A multistep approach in the cytologic evaluation of liver biopsy samples of dogs with hepatic diseases. *Vet. Pathol.* 41: 461–470.

19 Franceschini, B., Ceva-Grimaldi, G., Russo, C. et al. (2006). The complex functions of mast cells in chronic human liver diseases. *Dig. Dis. Sci.* 51: 2248–2256.

20 Fuentealba, C., Guest, S., Haywood, S., and Horney, B. (1997). Chronic hepatitis: a retrospective study in 34 dogs. *Can. Vet. J.* 38 (6): 365–373.

9

Cytological Features of Biliary Diseases

Biliary cells, which are always somewhat relegated to the back of the cytopathological scene (dominated by the hepatocytes), are very rarely found in a hepatic cytological sample. As already described in Chapter 2 on normal cytology, in my opinion, the main reason for this is the fact that small or large ductal structures are generally embedded in expanded bundles of fibrous connective tissue which, especially during pathological processes focused on the portal tract, tend to be abundant. According to the current standard, biliary diseases [1] are classified as follows.

- Ductal plate developmental disorders (biliary cystic diseases, congenital hepatic fibrosis, von Meyenburg complexes) and biliary atresia (congenital)
- Cholestasis and cholatestasis
- Cholangitis
- Gallbladder diseases

This list should also include those biliary diseases resulting from liver diseases (or which can be associated with liver diseases) that are not primarily biliary derived, such as some forms of chronic hepatitis, where bile duct hyperplasia can occur. Several forms of ductular reaction, described as the proliferation of reactive bile ducts, can be induced by liver inflammation [2].

Congenital ductal plate developmental disorders, resulting from embryonic development defects, can be found in various segments of the biliary tree. These disorders include **Caroli disease**, a condition affecting the largest branches of the bile duct, including the common bile duct and lobar ducts, producing cystic dilation. Other disorders affect the intermediate-sized bile ducts producing **congenital hepatic fibrosis** [3] and **polycystic disease of the adult**, which affects cats more frequently than dogs. Isolated ductal plate developmental anomalies of the small branches of the biliary tree lead to **von Meyenburg complexes**.

Canine and Feline Liver Cytology, First Edition. Carlo Masserdotti.
© 2024 John Wiley & Sons, Inc. Published 2024 by John Wiley & Sons, Inc.

Cytology alone is not able to recognize these pathological conditions, and a comprehensive explanation can be found in several specialized texts.

Cholestasis, a common pathological condition, very easily recognized cytologically, is the term used to refer to a disturbance in biliary outflow, associated with accumulation in the bloodstream of substances that are normally eliminated by the bile, such as bile acids, bilirubin or cholesterol.

Cytologically and histologically, bile accumulation, resulting from cholestasis, can produce casts or plugs of intensely basophilic dense material, found in canaliculi between hepatocytes. While this morphological aspect is difficult to evaluate in a histological sample, it is one of the cornerstones of cytological investigation, which is described in detail in Chapter 4. It is important to understand that it is cytologically impossible to establish the cause of cholestasis or to distinguish between conditions of extrahepatic or intrahepatic stasis. *Extrahepatic cholestasis* is caused by obstructive conditions to biliary outflow, including inflammation, stones, neoplasms, but also by obstructions induced by extrahepatic masses located near the great ducts, the gallbladder, the common duct and even in the duodenal papilla. *Intrahepatic cholestasis* is caused by conditions that prevent hepatocytes from excreting bile, including sepsis, drug- or toxin-induced injury or any injury to the hepatocytes, including hypoxia, as well as rare congenital conditions; swelling of hepatocytes, as in the case of severe steatosis, can also lead to intrahepatic cholestasis. A comprehensive evaluation of all the available data is necessary to properly determine the causes of cholestasis detected by cytological alterations.

Cholangitis, which can be either acute and chronic, is induced by primary or secondary inflammatory conditions. Acute forms of cholangitis, suppurative cholangitis induced by bacterial infections or destructive cholangitis caused by toxic, viral or pharmacological damage have no distinctive cytological features. Chronic cholangitis may lead to reactive biliary proliferation phenomena, and the cytological sample may contain sheets of biliary epithelium detached from the hyperplastic and replicated ducts.

Cytology can be helpful in the evaluation of pathological conditions that occur in bile or in the gallbladder. The morphological features of nonneoplastic and neoplastic conditions will be described in Chapter 12. Cytology of the bile is easy to perform, although mostly useful for inflammatory septic conditions. Gallbladder diseases are generally very difficult to investigate through cytological examination, mostly because of the cavitary nature of the organ and the technical difficulties of using a needle to sample parietal epithelium. Gallbladder diseases mainly involve inflammatory conditions, due to infection or neoplastic processes. Other diseases are caused by circulatory disorders, such as parietal necrosis induced by infarction or cystic mucinous hyperplasia of the gallbladder, which feature hyperplasia of the epithelium, with a substantial accumulation of mucinous material,

Table 9.1 Semiquantitative evaluation of the main cytological features of some biliary diseases.

	Bile casts	Number of cholangiocytes	Inflammatory cells
Acute cholestasis	+/++	−/+	−/+
Chronic cholestasis	+/++	+	−/+
Acute cholangitis	+/++	−	+/++
Chronic cholangitis	−/+	+/++	+/++
Lymphocytic cholangitis	−/+	+/++	+/+++

−: none; +: some; ++: moderate amount; +++: high amount.

which dilates the parietal epithelial structures and the lumen. This condition is well known in the clinical field for its characteristic and unmistakable ultrasound appearance [4].

Descriptions in the veterinary literature regarding the cytological criteria for the diagnosis of biliary diseases are quite rare and generally related to biliary neoplasms. Recently, I published an article dedicated to the cytological aspects of biliary diseases that has contributed to the identification of some morphological criteria. These criteria aid the identification of primary or secondary pathological processes [5]. The data obtained through this multi-year study can be used to shed light on the morphological aspects of this poorly understood area of hepatic cytology. In Table 9.1 a semiquantitive evaluation of the main cytological features of biliary diseases is represented.

9.1 General Features of Biliary Diseases

Cytomorphology: the biliary elements exfoliate, in pathological conditions, mostly from small ducts and are represented by cells smaller than hepatocytes, with cuboidal, weakly basophilic cytoplasm and a round granular or compact chromatin nucleus, organized in variably cohesive, bi- or three-dimensional strips, sometimes in rows or palisade arrangements (Figure 9.1). There may be achromatic cytoplasmic microglobules, with nonspecific significance, perhaps related to metabolic diseases such as diabetes or hyperplastic phenomena (Figure 9.2). It is important to remember that, in this context, bile cells must be differentiated from aggregates of mesothelial elements coming from the Glisson's capsule.

The presence of bile epithelium in a hepatic cytological sample is always an unusual event (Figure 9.3). The presence of cholangiocytes in a cytological sample should always be interpreted as a pathological marker, especially when there are

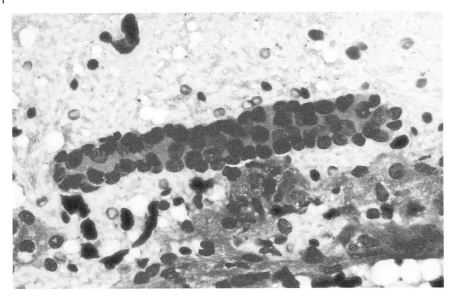

Figure 9.1 Liver, chronic cholangitis, FNCS, dog. The presence of biliary cells, represented by cuboidal cells with bluish cytoplasm and round nuclei with granular to compact chromatin, is a rare finding, even when a biliary disease exists (MGG, 100×).

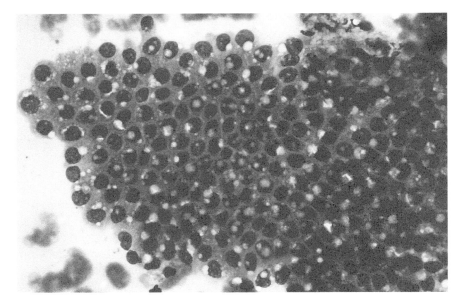

Figure 9.2 Liver, chronic cholangitis and diabetes, FNCS, dog. The presence of small achromatic globules inside the cytoplasm of cholangiocytes is an aspecific finding, sometimes related to metabolic conditions (MGG, 100×).

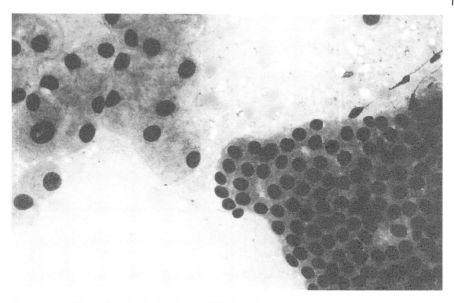

Figure 9.3 Liver, chronic cholangitis, FNCS, dog. The presence of large clusters of cholangiocytes should always be interpreted as a pathological change, mostly related to a primary or secondary cholangiopathy (MGG, 100×).

clinical, laboratory, and ultrasound alterations compatible with a disorder of the bile ducts. Unfortunately, in most cases, it is difficult to collect sufficient morphological data for a definitive diagnosis and, as in several other pathological conditions of the liver, the findings must be treated with caution and should be followed by histopathological evaluation.

9.2 Cytological Features of Specific Biliary Diseases

9.2.1 Acute and Chronic Cholestasis

Cytomorphology: casts of bile material between the hepatocytes; during acute cholestasis, presence of very rare aggregates consisting of cholangiocytes with cuboidal cytoplasm, as well as weakly basophilic and round nuclei, with granular or compact chromatin (Figure 9.4). During chronic cholestasis, large aggregates of cholangiocytes may be observed, sometimes with honeycomb arrangement (Figure 9.5); palisade arrangements may be also seen. Chronic cholestasis may be associated with cytological findings indicating fibrosis and nonspecific hepatocellular damage (Figure 9.6).

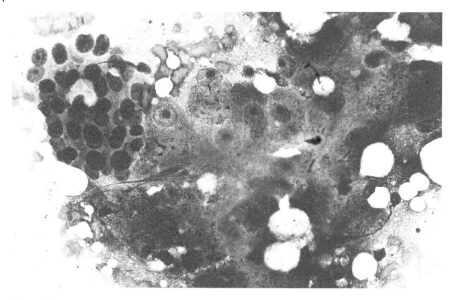

Figure 9.4 Liver, acute cholestasis, FNCS, dog. In acute cholestasis, as well as the presence of casts of biliary material among the hepatocytes, it is possible to observe, in very rare cases, small clusters of cholangiocytes (MGG, 100×).

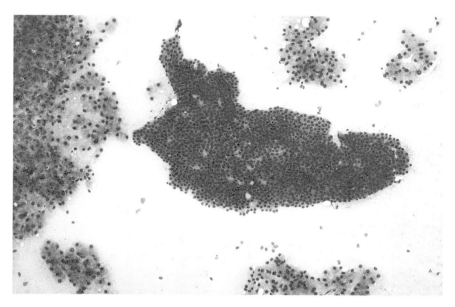

Figure 9.5 Liver, chronic cholestasis, FNCS, dog. The presence of large clusters of cholangiocytes, although an inconstant finding, may be related to hepatic diseases with chronic cholestasis; notice the honeycomb arrangement among cholangiocytes (MGG, 40×).

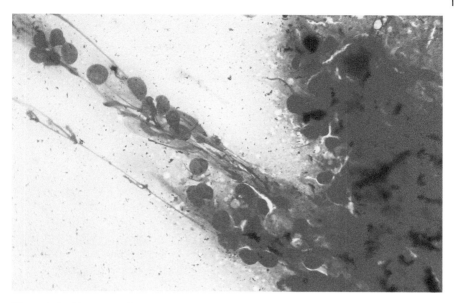

Figure 9.6 Liver, chronic cholestasis, FNCS, dog. Cholestasis may be present together with fibrosis and hepatocellular reversible injury (MGG, 100×).

As described in Chapter 4 on extracytoplasmic pathological accumulations, the morphological criterion indicating cholestasis is the presence of casts of bile material between the hepatocytes. In cases of acute cholestasis, it is very difficult to see cholangiocytes on cytology, probably because the pathological event did not have sufficient time to induce proliferation of the cholangiocytes. Indeed, histologically, acute cholestasis is characterized by portal tract edema and inflammatory cells, typically neutrophils and sometimes disruption of the biliary ducts [1]. In contrast, in the course of chronic cholestasis, the event that caused the stasis of the bile outflow may persist long enough to allow replication of the ducts; sheets of cholangiocytes with a moderate to high number of cholangiocytes were observed in 47.6% of dogs and 32% of cats with chronic cholestasis [5]. The reason why biliary cells are an inconstant finding in chronic cholesatasis is the fact that proliferated ducts are embedded in abundant connective tissue, making exfoliation more difficult.

The main causes of cholestasis have been discussed in Chapter 4, which should be consulted for further information. The clinical conditions that can induce acute cholestasis include so-called "destructive cholangitis" of smaller and distal portal tracts. This condition is generally induced by an adverse response to drugs, viral infections (distemper), and toxic damage. Despite being rare, these conditions can determine an acute bile stasis which, in severe cases, may even cause the emission of acolytic stools.

9.2.2   Acute Cholangitis

Cytomorphology: nonspecific and reversible damage to hepatocytes, presence of bile casts among the hepatocytes. Biliary epithelial cells are normally not detected, but in some cases inflammatory elements may be found, especially neutrophilic granulocytes with karyolytic appearance. Occasionally, phagocytosis of bacteria is evident.

Acute cholangitis is a fairly rare condition mostly affecting cats, which originates from ascending infections from the intestine or possibly the systemic circulation. Biliary exfoliation cannot be detected, as pathological processes of this type are mainly represented by periductal edema and neutrophilic inflammatory infiltration which are nonspecific in a cytological sample, unless they show karyolysis and possibly bacterial phagocytosis. In the course of acute processes, the biliary epithelium does not normally expand, so the detection of cholangiocytes is highly unlikely. Similarly to what was previously described, the condition known as destructive cholangitis of the smaller and distal portal tracts can be associated with loss of biliary tract and inflammatory infiltration caused by macrophages and neutrophils.

9.2.3   Chronic Cholangitis

Cytomorphology: presence of biliary epithelial aggregates, generally represented by cells with weakly basophilic and indistinct cuboidal cytoplasm, sometimes filled with small achromatic globules containing a slightly dismetric round nucleus, with granular or compact chromatin (Figure 9.7). Bile casts may be detected among the hepatocytes, that may be affected by nonspecific and reversible hepatocellular damage. Sometimes, variable fibrosis and mixed inflammation are present (Figure 9.8); inflammation, mostly in subacute conditions or when secondary bacterial infection occurs, may be represented by neutrophilic granulocytes. The presence of bacteria is an inconstant finding (Figures 9.9–9.11).

Aggregated cholangiocytes may be observed in canine and feline cases, respectively in 63.5% and 52.4%. Similarly to other forms of chronic cholangitis, this pathological process affecting the biliary tract may cause abundant exfoliation of cholangiocytes.

In conclusion, producing a cytological diagnosis of chronic cholangitis is virtually impossible, but the evidence of said morphological features should prompt the clinician to perform a histological investigation.

9.2.4   Lymphocytic Cholangitis

Cytomorphology: exfoliation of a moderate number of biliary sheets, sometimes represented by a large number of cells, without specific alterations is an inconstant finding (Figure 9.12); a variable number of small and intermediate,

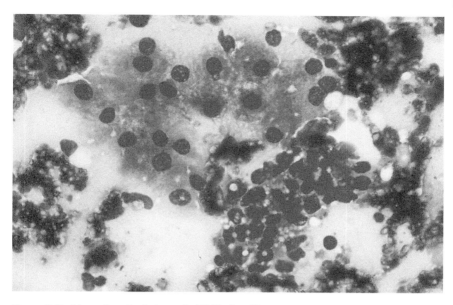

Figure 9.7   Liver, chronic cholestasis, FNCS, dog. The presence of cholangiocytes in small to medium-sized aggregates is an inconstant finding; notice the small achromatic globules inside the cytoplasm of cholangiocytes (MGG, 100×).

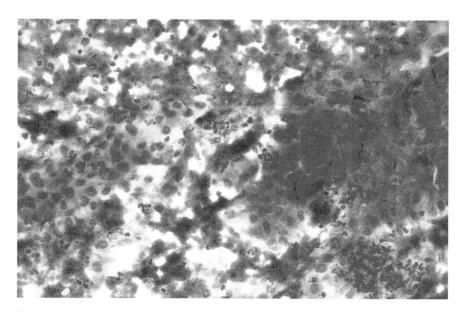

Figure 9.8   Liver, chronic cholestasis, FNCS, dog. In chronic cholangitis, small to medium-sized clusters of cholangiocytes, inflammatory cells, and hepatocytes may be a diagnostic finding (MGG, 100×).

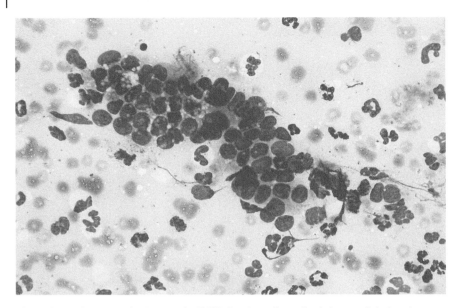

Figure 9.9 Liver, chronic cholestasis, FNCS, dog. A medium-sized cluster of cholangiocytes surrounded by well-preserved to degenerate neutrophilic granulocytes. Notice, at the top, two neutrophils that phagocytize small coccoid and rod-to-filamentous bacteria (MGG, 100×).

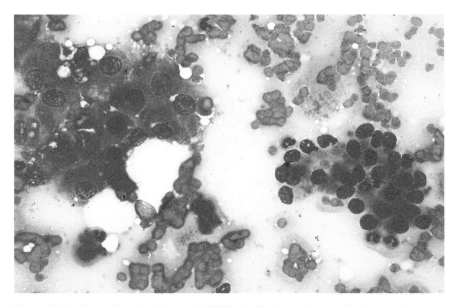

Figure 9.10 Liver, chronic cholestasis, FNCS, dog. To the right, a small cluster of cholangiocytes; notice the neutrophilic granulocytes that surround or infiltrate the aggregate (MGG, 100×).

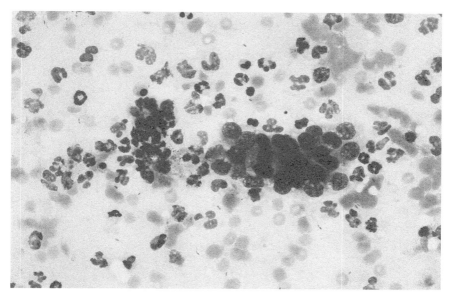

Figure 9.11 Liver, chronic cholestasis, FNCS, dog. Bacteria may be observed on the background, here associated with many well-preserved to degenerate neutrophils and a small cluster of cholangiocytes (MGG, 100×).

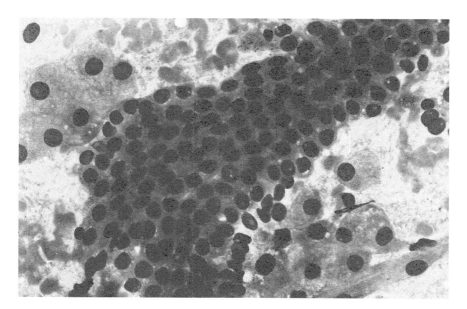

Figure 9.12 Liver, lymphocytic cholangitis, FNCS, cat. In very rare cases of lymphocytic cholangitis, large aggregate of cholangiocytes may exfoliate near to hepatocytes (MGG, 100×).

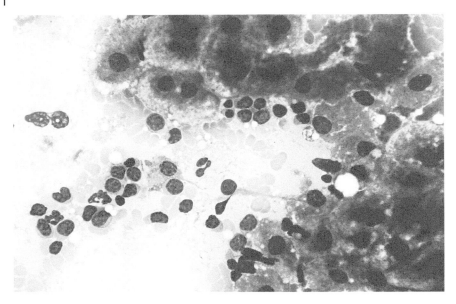

Figure 9.13 Liver, lymphocytic cholangitis, FNCS, cat. Small to medium-sized lymphocytes in variable numbers may be observed scattered around the hepatocytes or on the background (MGG, 100×).

sometimes large lymphocytes and rare plasma cells, which may concentrate in the proximity of the cholangiocyte aggregates. The lymphocytes may be concentrated around hepatocytes (Figure 9.13), affected by reversible nonspecific damage (especially lipidosis), while cholestasis and fibrosis are less likely.

This disease has been widely described in cats while in dogs it is extremely rare (one case out of 58, 1.9% of cholangitis) [6]. This disease is also referred to as "lymphocytic cholangiohepatitis," "lymphocytic portal hepatitis" or "nonsuppurative cholangitis" [7–9]; recently, as cholangitis progresses as a continuum to cholangiohepatitis, the term "nonsuppurative cholangitis-cholangiohepatitis" has been proposed [10].

The etiology of this condition is virtually unknown, although immune-mediated mechanisms seem to be the most likely cause [11]. Hypothetically, an ascending bacterial infection could initiate an inflammatory process, generally represented by neutrophilic cholangitis that, by chronicization, could trigger an immune-mediated process in which lymphocytes predominate. Ascending bacterial infection can be the consequence of extrahepatic conditions including pancreatic, gastrointestinal, and, to a lesser degree, renal diseases [12]. Moreover lymphocytic cholangitis may be associated with pancreatitis and chronic enteritis, a combination known as "triaditis" [13], resulting from a reflux of enteric bacteria that ascend the common duct. Nevertheless, although chronic inflammation can be sustained as immune-mediated disease after the etiological agent has been eliminated, recent evidence does not support a role for bacteria in the etiopathogenesis of lymphocytic cholangitis, but rather suggests an immune-mediated mechanism [10, 14]. Advanced and chronic stages are frequently associated with ductal proliferation and fibrosis, with the latter varying considerably [10].

The main differential diagnosis for lymphocytic cholangitis, particularly in cats, is lymphoma. Given the high number and small size of lymphocytes, the possibility of a small cell lymphoma is a concern. In addition to cytology or histology, other in-depth investigations aimed at excluding lymphoma are often required, such as immunohistochemistry and clonality evaluations by polymerase chain reaction (PCR) for antigen receptor rearrangement (PARR) [10].

9.3 Key Points

- Biliary cells are generally not present in a cytological sample; when sheets of cholangiocytes are detected, a cholangiopathy should be suspected.
- Cholangiocytes are easily distinguished from hepatocytes, by the small cuboidal cytoplasm and the round nucleus with compact to granular chromatin; cholangiocytes also occur in tight packed sheets. Care must be taken in differentiate cholangiocytes from mesothelial cells.
- The number of cholangiocytes in samples from liver affected by a cholangiopathy is highly variable.
- The likelihood of correctly recognizing a specific type of cholangiopathy is low and a comparison with all the clinical, laboratory, and ultrasonographic data is always warranted.
- Although cytology is frequently able to provide data that allow recognition of a cholangiopathy, histological evaluation is always necessary for a definitive diagnosis.

References

1 Van den Ingh, T.S.G.A.M., Cullen, J.M., Twedt, D.C. et al. (2006). Morphological classification of biliary disorders of the canine and feline liver. In: *Standard for Clinical and Histological Diagnosis of Canine and Feline Liver Disease* (ed. WSAVA Liver Standardization Group), 61–76. St Louis, MO: Saunders.

2 Sato, K., Marzioni, M., Meng, F. et al. (2019). Ductular reaction in liver diseases: pathological mechanisms and translational significances. *Hepatology* 69 (1): 420–430.

3 Brown, D.L., van Winkle, T., Cecere, T. et al. (2010). Congenital hepatic fibrosis in 5 dogs. *Vet. Pathol.* 47 (1): 102–107.

4 Besso, J.G., Wrigley, R.H., Gliatto, J.M., and Webster, C.R. (2000). Ultrasonographic appearance and clinical findings in 14 dogs with galladder mucus. *Vet. Radiol. Ultrasound* 41 (3): 261–271.

5 Masserdotti, C. (2020). The cytologic features of biliary diseases: a retrospective study. *Vet. Clin. Pathol.* 49 (3): 440–450.

6 Harrison, J.L., Turek, B.J., Brown, D.C. et al. (2018). Cholangitis and cholangiohepatitis in dogs: a descriptive study of 54 cases based on histopathologic diagnosis (2004–2014). *J. Vet. Intern. Med.* 32 (1): 172–180.

7 Day, D.G. (1995). Feline cholangiohepatitis complex. *Vet. Clin. North Am. Small Anim. Pract.* 25 (2): 375–385.

8 Gagne, J.M., Weiss, D.J., and Armstrong, P.J. (1996). Histopathologic evaluation of feline inflammatory liver disease. *Vet. Pathol.* 33 (5): 521–526.

9 Weiss, D.J., Armstrong, P.J., and Gagne, J.M. (1997). Inflammatory liver disease. *Semin. Vet. Med. Surg. Small Anim.* 12 (1): 22–27.

10 Warren, A., Center, S., McDonough, S. et al. (2011). Histopathologic features, immunophenotyping, clonality, and eubacterial fluorescence in situ hybridization in cats with lymphocytic cholangitis/cholangiohepatitis. *Vet. Pathol.* 48 (3): 627–641.

11 Boland, L. and Beatty, J. (2017). Feline cholangitis. *Vet. Clin. North Am. Small Anim. Pract.* 47 (3): 703–724.

12 Weiss, D.J., Gagne, J.M., and Armstrong, J. (1996). Relationship between inflammatory hepatic disease and inflammatory bowel disease, pancreatitis, and nephritis in cats. *J. Am. Vet. Med. Assoc.* 209: 1114–1116.

13 Simpson, K.W. (2015). Pancreatitis and triaditis in cats: causes and treatment. *J. Small Anim. Pract.* 56 (1): 40–49.

14 Clark, J.E.C., Haddad, J.L., Brown, D.C. et al. (2011). Feline cholangitis: a necropsy study of 44 cats (1986–2008). *J. Feline Med. Surg.* 13 (8): 570–576.

10

Bile and Gallbladder Diseases

Bile is the main product of the liver, produced by the hepatocytes, stored in the gallbladder and discharged into the intestine, mostly with an emulsificatory role enhancing digestion of alimentary lipids. The bile is composed of a mixture of water, bile salts, metabolites such as bilirubin, lipids (cholesterol, fatty acids), xenobiotic conjugates, inorganic salts, and lysosomal debris together with antibodies and cytokines. An evaluation of bile in normal conditions is only possible by fine needle aspiration of the gallbladder.

The gallbladder, also known as the cholecyst, is a hollow organ where bile is stored and concentrated before it is released into the duodenum. The gallbladder wall is composed of an epithelium, lamina propria, and a fibromuscular layer. The epithelium is thrown into folds, arranged in low papillary projections; columnar epithelial cells produce mucus and absorb or secrete substances; the fibromuscular layer may contract and facilitate the flow of bile; the blood supply is limited to an artery derived from the left hepatic artery.

Normal bile from the gallbladder grossly appears as dense, dark-green-to-yellowish-brown fluid; after a smear is made, with Romanowsky staining, bile appears as blue to green-gray granular, amorphous to wispy material (Figure 10.1); the same material may appear in large clumps (Figure 10.2). Occasional columnar cells from the epithelium may exfoliate on the background [1].

A lot of gallbladder diseases [2, 3], including traumatic diseases, cholecystitis, cholelithiasis, necrotizing cholecystitis, consequences of pancreatitis (mostly in cat), mucoceles and neoplasms, are evaluable on the basis of historical, clinical, clinicopathological, and ultrasonographic examination [4]. Histopathology is necessary to diagnose neutrophilic and lymphoplasmacytic cholecystitis [5]. The diagnosis of infarction and neoplastic diseases also requires histological evaluation. Cytological examination of bile may be helpful in the evaluation of inflammatory diseases, to confirm the diagnosis of mucocele and in evaluation of some neoplasms.

Canine and Feline Liver Cytology, First Edition. Carlo Masserdotti.

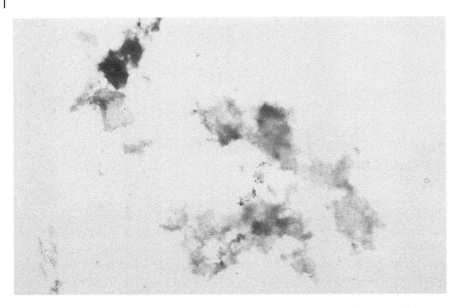

Figure 10.1 Normal bile, flushing, dog. On a clean background, the biliary material sometimes aggregates in small, loose clumps (MGG, 100×).

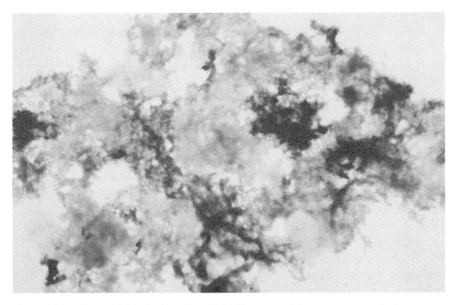

Figure 10.2 Normal bile, flushing, dog. The biliary material may aggregate in large, basophilic clumps of amorphous material (MGG, 100×).

10.1 Bactibilia and Septic Cholecystitis

Cytomorphology: presence of coccoid, rod-shaped or filamentous organisms (Figure 10.3); number may be extremely variable, on a blue to green-gray granular, amorphous to wispy background. When luminal inflammation is present, degenerate neutrophils may show phagocytosis of bacteria (Figure 10.4) along with a variable amount of debris and inspissated basophilic material.

Cytological examination of bile, complemented by aerobic and anaerobic bacterial culture results, is helpful in detecting the presence of bacteria [6]; also, with or without inflammatory cells, it can led to a clinical decision to initiate antimicrobial treatment. Furthermore, cytology and culture of the bile are very useful for antimicrobial treatment monitoring [7, 8].

Cases with apparent negative bacterial culture resulting in the presence of bacteria detected in cytological specimens have been described [9]. In these cases, if the patient is symptomatic for bacterial infection, laboratory changes are consistent with bacterial cholangitis, or ultrasonographic changes are detected, empirical antibiotic therapy, based on bacteria seen on cytology, may be the correct clinical choice, as previous antibiotic therapy may impair the ability of bacteria to grow in culture.

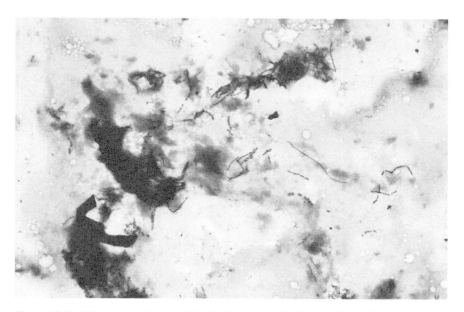

Figure 10.3   Bile, chronic cholecystitis, flushing, dog. Bile is normally sterile; the presence of bacteria scattered on the background, although not definitively diagnostic, may be associated with cholecystitis or cholangitis (MGG, 100×).

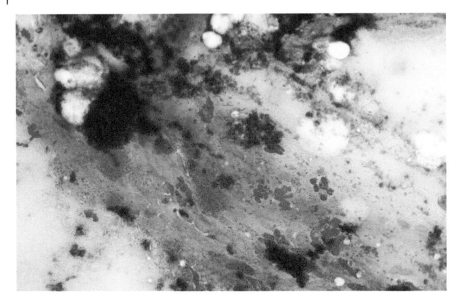

Figure 10.4   Bile, acute, neutrophilic, septic cholecystitis, flushing, dog. The presence of degenerate neutrophilic granulocytes that phagocytize bacteria, also present on the background, is diagnostic for septic cholecystitis, possibly associated with cholangitis (MGG, 100×).

Bile culture alone, without cytological examination, may not be diagnostically accurate, as protozoal and others bacterial organisms could be missed. *Escherichia coli*, *Enterococcus* spp., *Bacteroides* spp., *Streptococcus* spp., and *Clostridium* spp. were the most common true-positive isolates [10]. Antimicrobial resistance of aerobic isolates in dogs has been reported in only one study so far [11].

Other than bacteria, other microorganisms can be detectable in bile. *Cyniclomyces guttulatus*, a fungal microorganism, was observed in a dog with bactibilia, probably as an incidental finding [12].

Large, yellow-brown, oval structures measuring approximately 40–45 × 25–30 μm are the eggs of *Platynosomum fastosum*, a trematode inhabiting the hepatobiliary tract of domestic cats. Karyolytic, pyknotic, and karyorrhectic neutrophils have been described in the bile from a cat from Florida [13].

Small, crescent-shaped organisms, approximately 4–5 μm in length and 0.5 μm in width, with smooth, brightly basophilic cytoplasm and oval-shaped nuclei, oriented parallel to the long axis, recognized as Sarcocystidae micro0rganisms, were found on the bile smears of a dog with acute hepatitis [14].

10.2   Epithelial Hyperplasia

Cytomorphology: variable number of columnar cells with mild anisokaryosis and anisocytosis, in bi- or tridimensional clusters, with palisade arrangement may be evident on a blue to green-gray granular, amorphous to wispy basophilic background (Figure 10.5).

In cases of subacute to chronic inflammatory diseases of the gallbladder, the epithelium may undergo reactive, hyperplastic changes [15]. Care must be taken not to confuse the hyperplastic epithelium with a neoplastic process; in this distinction, the support of ultrasonographic examination is mandatory.

10.3   Gallbladder Mucocele

Cytomorphology: exfoliation of abundant, dispersed or thickened eosinophilic or basophilic mucous material (Figure 10.6), on which it is possible to detect cell debris, rare leukocytes, occasionally aggregates of basophilic cytoplasmic columnar bile cells and round basal nucleus, with granular or compact chromatin.

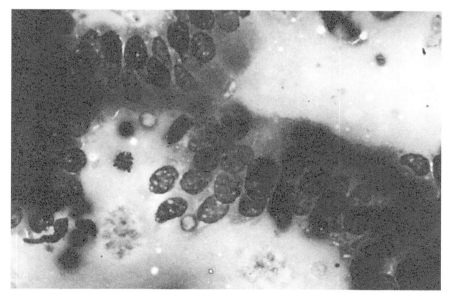

Figure 10.5   Bile, chronic hyperplastic cholecystitis, flushing, dog. A large cluster of columnar epithelial cells on the surface of the gallbladder (MGG, 100×).

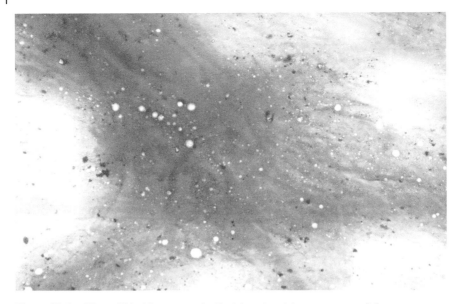

Figure 10.6 Bile, gallbladder mucocele, flushing, dog. A large amount of dense eosinophilic material may be sampled in cases of gallbladder mucocele (MGG, 100×).

Gallbladder mucocele (GBM) is an abnormal, intraluminal accumulation of inspissated, semisolid bile and/or mucus within the gallbladder, probably related to changes in the biophysical structure of proteins, altering the physical and functional properties of mucus produced by the parietal cells [16]. The etiology is unknown but risk factors include hyperadrenocorticism, hypothyroidism, dyslipidemia, or use of some drugs such as thyroxine or imidacloprid [17]. A mutation in the ABCB4 gene has been considered a risk factor, since it may be associated with a decrease of phospholipid concentration in the biliary lumen and increased cytotoxicity of bile salts; however, recent studies seem to exclude an association between mutation and GBM [18]. The relevant bibliography suggests correlations with breed and consequently with familial or genetic causes [19, 20].

Clinical signs, when present, are often nonspecific, including vomiting, lethargy, anorexia, abdominal pain, and polydipsia-polyuria; the results of complete blood count are unremarkable, although leukocytosis with left shift neutrophils was evident in 46.9% of cases [21]. Also an increase in liver enzymes, including alanine aminotransferase (87.4% of cases), aspartate aminotransferase (62.2%), alkaline phosphatase (98.2%) and gamma-glutamyltransferase (85.7%), may be detected [2]. Although icterus is present in approximately 16.3% of cases [22], hyperbilirubinemia is reported in significantly more instances (83.2%) [2]. Cystic mucinous hyperplasia of the gallbladder, especially when involving the large ducts adjacent to the gallbladder, or extrusion of mucus could obstruct biliary outflow, resulting in cholestasis. In addition, mucocele could create the conditions for the development of chronic cholangitis or necrosis of the gallbladder wall, with rupture and choleperitoneum.

Sampling of the accumulated material, via needle aspiration, may be clinically necessary to evaluate dilation of the gallbladder, especially if septic inflammatory conditions are considered to be likely.

10.4   Limy Bile Syndrome

Recently, limy bile syndrome, a rare entity in which there is an excessive precipitation of calcium salts, mainly calcium carbonate in the gallbladder and to a rare extent in the common bile duct, has been described in a dog. The gallbladder can be filled with a semisolid, paste-like greenish-brown material composed of 80% calcium carbonate, consistent with the so-called "limy bile" [23].

10.5   Biliary Sludge

Biliary sludge is a dense, viscous mixture of cholesterol crystals, calcium products, mucin, and other materials resulting from delayed excretion [24, 25]. Since biliary sludge may be associated with gallbladder dysmotility and mucus hypersecretion, a link between biliary sludge and the formation of gallbladder mucocele has been suggested [26]. Cytological examination is a reliable diagnostic method to confirm the ultrasonographic diagnosis [27]. On cytological examination of the bile, the presence of microspheroliths, represented by yellow-brown crystals likely composed of calcium carbonate, sometimes admixed with mucoid, blue-gray material, is evident (Figure 10.7).

10.6   Neoplastic Diseases of Gallbladder

Benign and malignant neoplasms may originate in the epithelium or the wall of the gallbladder. Biliary carcinoma, neuroendocrine tumors, stromal tumors, and hematoma have been described. Cytological descriptions of some neoplasms will be given in Chapter 12.

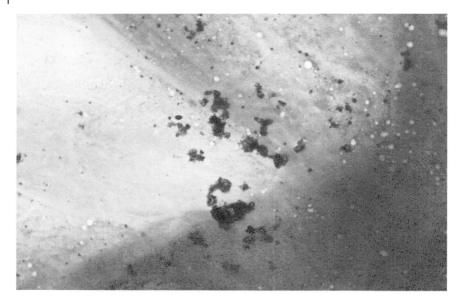

Figure 10.7 Bile, biliary sludge, flushing, dog. Yellow-brown crystals are present on a dense, eosinophilic background (MGG, 100×).

10.7 Other Gallbladder Diseases

Gallstones [28], with or without obstruction, wall infarct [29], and edema [30] are uncommon diseases that are not evaluable by cytology alone.

10.8 Key Points

- Cytological evaluation of the bile is a useful diagnostic method, mostly in recognition of inflammatory septic diseases.
- Many diseases of the gallbladder are not evaluable by cytology, since the thin wall is frequently not a target for needle sampling.
- Cytology may be useful in diagnosis of neoplastic diseases, in cases where a mass is present in the wall of the gallbladder.

References

1 Flatland, B. (2009). If you have the gall... . *Vet. Clin. Pathol.* 38: 280.
2 Center, S.A. (2009). Diseases of the gallbladder and biliary tree. *Vet. Clin. North Am. Small Anim. Pract.* 39 (3): 543–598.

3 Neer, T.M. (1992). A review of disorders of the gallbladder and extrahepatic biliary tract in the dog and cat. *J. Vet. Intern. Med.* 6 (3): 186–192.

4 Brand, E.M., Lim, C.K., Heng, H.G. et al. (2020). Computed tomographic features of confirmed gallbladder pathology in 34 dogs. *Vet. Radiol. Ultrasound* 61 (6): 667–679.

5 Harrison, J.L., Turek, B.J., Brown, D.C. et al. (2018). Cholangitis and cholangiohepatitis in dogs: a descriptive study of 54 cases based on histopathologic diagnosis (2004–2014). *J. Vet. Intern. Med.* 32 (1): 172–180.

6 Ramery, E., Papakonstantinou, S., Pinilla, M. et al. (2012). Bacterial cholangiohepatitis in a dog. *Can. Vet. J.* 53 (4): 423–425.

7 Peters, L.M., Glanemann, B., Garden, O.A., and Szladovits, B. (2016). Cytological findings of 140 bile samples from dogs and cats and associated clinical pathological data. *J. Vet. Intern. Med.* 30: 123–131.

8 Ruaux, C.G., Nemanic, S., and Milovancev, M. (2015). Characterization, treatment, and outcome of bacterial cholecystitis and bactibilia in dogs. *J. Am. Vet. Med. Assoc.* 246: 982–989.

9 Pashmakova, M.B., Piccione, J., Bishop, M.A. et al. (2017). Agreement between microscopic examination and bacterial culture of bile samples for detection of bactibilia in dogs and cats with hepatobiliary disease. *J. Am. Vet. Med. Assoc.* 250 (9): 1007–1013.

10 Wagner, K.A., Hartmann, F.A., and Trepanier, L.A. (2007). Bacterial culture results from liver, gallbladder, or bile in 248 dogs and cats evaluated for hepatobiliary disease: 1998–2003. *J. Vet. Intern. Med.* 21 (3): 417–424.

11 Tamborini, A., Jahns, H., McAllister, H. et al. (2016). Bacterial cholangitis, cholecystitis, or both in dogs. *J. Vet. Intern. Med.* 30: 1046–1055.

12 Neel, J.A., Tarigo, J., and Grindem, C.B. (2006). Gallbladder aspirate from a dog. *Vet. Clin. Pathol.* 35 (4): 467–470.

13 Stern, J.K., Walden, H.D.S., Marshall, K., and Sharkey, L. (2020). What is your diagnosis? Bile from a cat. *Vet. Clin. Pathol.* 49 (2): 354–355.

14 Irvine, K.L., Walker, J.M., and Friedrichs, K.R. (2016). Sarcocystid organisms found in bile from a dog with acute hepatitis: a case report and review of intestinal and hepatobiliary Sarcocystidae infections in dogs and cats. *Vet. Clin. Pathol.* 45 (1): 57–65.

15 Miyano, T., Tokumaru, T., Suzuki, F., and Suda, K. (1989). Adenoma and stone formation of the biliary tract in puppies that had choledochopancreatic anastomosis. *J. Pediatr. Surg.* 24 (6): 539–542.

16 Kesimer, M., Cullen, J.M., Cao, R. et al. (2015). Excess secretion of gel-forming mucins and associated innate defense proteins with defective mucin un-packaging underpin gallbladder mucocele formation in dogs. *PLoS One* 10 (9): e0138988.

17 Gookin, L., Correa, M.T., Peters, A. et al. (2015). Association of gallbladder mucocele histologic diagnosis with selected drug use in dogs: a matched case-control study. *J. Vet. Intern. Med.* 29 (6): 1464–1472.

18 Cullen, J.M., Willson, C.J., Minch, J.D. et al. (2014). Lack of association of ABCB4 oc insertion mutation with gallbladder mucoceles in dogs. *J. Vet. Diagn. Invest.* 26 (3): 434–436.

19 Aguirre, A.L., Center, S.A., Randolph, J.F. et al. (2007). Gallbladder disease in Shetland sheepdogs: 38 cases (1995–2005). *J. Am. Vet. Med. Assoc.* 231 (1): 79–88.

20 Malek, S., Sinclair, E., Hosgood, G. et al. (2013). Clinical findings and prognostic factors for dogs undergoing cholecystectomy for gall bladder mucocele. *Vet. Surg.* 42 (4): 418–426.

21 Worley, D.R., Hottinger, H.A., and Lawrence, H.J. (2004). Surgical management of gallbladder mucoceles in dogs: 22 cases (1999–2003). *J. Am. Vet. Med. Assoc.* 225 (9): 1418–1422.

22 Pike, F.S., Berg, J., King, N.W. et al. (2004). Gallbladder mucocele in dogs: 30 cases (2000–2002). *J. Am. Vet. Med. Assoc.* 224 (10): 1615–1622.

23 Fabrès, V., Layssol-Lamour, C., Meynaud-Collard, P., and Dossin, O. (2020). Limy bile syndrome in a dog. *J. Small Anim. Pract.* 61 (2): 137–140.

24 Peters, L.M. and Meyer, D.J. (2023). Hepatobiliary system. In: *Canine and Feline Cytopathology*, 4e (ed. R.E. Raskin, D.J. Meyer, and K.M. Boes), 339–376. St Louis, MO: Elsevier.

25 Tsukagoshi, T., Ohno, K., Tsukamoto, A. et al. (2012). Decreased gallbladder emptying in dogs with biliary sludge or gallbladder mucocele. *Vet. Radiol. Ultrasound* 53 (1): 84–91.

26 DeMonaco, S.M., Grant, D.C., Larson, M.M. et al. (2016). Spontaneous course of biliary sludge over 12 months in dogs with ultrasonographically identified biliary sludge. *J. Vet. Intern. Med.* 30 (3): 771–778.

27 Cook, A.K., Jambhekar, A.V., and Dylewski, A.M. (2016). Gallbladder sludge in dogs: ultrasonographic and clinical findings in 200 patients. *J. Am. Anim. Hosp. Assoc.* 52 (3): 125–131.

28 Cullen, J.M. and Stalker, M.J. (2016). Liver and biliary system. In: *Jubb, Kennedy and Palmer's Pathology of Domestic Animals*, VIe (ed. M.G. Maxie), 310–311. St Louis, MO: Elsevier.

29 Holt, D.E., Mehler, S., Mayhew, P.D., and Hendrick, M.J. (2004). Canine gallbladder infarction: 12 cases (1993–2003). *Vet. Pathol.* 41 (4): 416–418.

30 Lisciandro, G.R., Gambino, J.M., and Lisciandro, S.C. (2021). Thirteen dogs and a cat with ultrasonographically detected gallbladder wall edema associated with cardiac disease. *J. Vet. Intern. Med.* 35 (3): 1342–1346.

11

Etiological Agents

Cytology is, in my view, the best method for direct observation of microorganisms and, on the basis of associated inflammation, recognition of their pathological role in a tissue. Compared with histology, cytology is much more effective in recognition of viruses, bacteria, fungi, and some parasites because of the high definition of shape and size of microorganisms with standard stains. Moreover, in cases in which recognition is unclear, some special stains can be easily performed on cytological samples as confirmation; for example, Ziehl–Neelsen stain can help to confirm the presence of *Mycobacterium* spp. and periodic acid-Schiff (PAS) stain can be used in identification of fungi.

Nevertheless, to correctly diagnose a pathological process, where microorganisms and inflammatory cells are evident, it is advisable to compare the cytological features with the histological sample, mostly to establish if the inflammatory process is primary or secondary to other conditions: Chapter 6 on inflammation describes the limits of inflammatory cells in a cytological sample. Moreover, when an inflammatory population suggests the role of a microorganism in the pathological process, a definitive diagnosis often requires confirmation with microbiological methods [1], particularly if it is necessary to know the name of the bacterial or fungal agent and its responsiveness to antibiotic therapy.

As the recipient of both the portal and systemic circulation, the liver plays an important role in host defense against invasive microorganisms. Since Kupffer cells are involved in defense against liver infections, compromised anatomy or cell function results in impaired clearance and is alleged to be a predisposing event that facilitates bacterial invasion into the hepatic parenchyma [2]. Consequently, many cases of primary liver disease may be due to microorganism invasion – microrganisms may ascend the duodenal papilla from the intestinal lumen and invade the liver through the biliary tree.

The detection of a microorganism in a cytological sample must be compared with other changes, such as inflammation, phagocytosis from neutrophils and

Canine and Feline Liver Cytology, First Edition. Carlo Masserdotti.
© 2024 John Wiley & Sons, Inc. Published 2024 by John Wiley & Sons, Inc.

macrophages, reversible or irreversible changes of hepatocytes and cholangio-cytes, extensive necrosis or fibrosis, in order to correctly interpretate the patho-logical process.

11.1 Viruses

Cytomorphology: canine adenovirus-1 appears as dense, homogeneous, irregu-larly rounded eosinophilic bodies of variable size (Figure 11.1), sometimes sur-rounded by a thin area of marginated chromatin, visibly different from the nucleolus, which is generally small or inconsistent and always basophilic. They may be associated with nonspecific hepatocellular damage and inflammatory conditions.

While viruses can infect the liver, cytology has limited potential for diagnosis. Canine infectious hepatitis caused by canine adenovirus-1 is probably the only detectable virus in liver [3]. Other viral agents demonstrated or suspected to be causes of hepatic disease include Herpesvirus [4] and canine Bocavirus, classified as a genus within the Parvoviridae family [5]. Canine Circovirus has been isolated

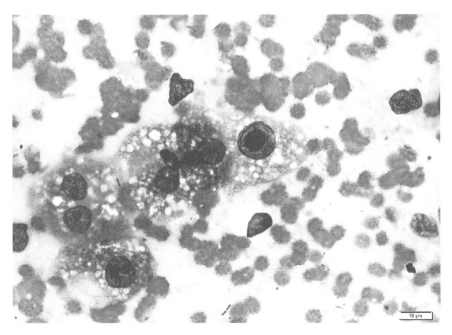

Figure 11.1 Liver, adenovirus hepatitis, FNCS, dog. Viral inclusion, represented by a large, deeply eosinophilic body inside the nucleus (MGG, 100×). *Source:* Courtesy of Dr Marian Taulescu.

from the liver of dogs and, from the same animals, viral cytoplasmic inclusions have been observed in macrophages [6].

11.2 Bacteria

Bacteria most frequently associated with hepatitis include *E.coli*, *Streptococcus* spp., *Staphylococcus* spp., *Enterococcus* spp., and *Clostridium* spp. [7]. The role of cytology is mostly to help in recognizing the coccoid (Figure 11.2), rod-shaped (Figure 11.3) or filamentous bacteria (Figures 11.4 and 11.5) and their phagocytosis from neutrophils and macrophages, and to provide valuable help in establishing the presence of a primary or secondary infectious disease. Other bacteria are recognized as causative agents of hepatic disease, such as *Leptospira* spp. and *Helicobacter* spp. (Figure 11.6), although cytology is not able to detect these and culture is often required to identify organisms [8–10]. *Mycobacterium* spp. can cause hepatic disease (Figure 11.7); organisms appear as small nonstaining rods in the cytoplasm of activated macrophages [11], sometimes in high numbers (Figure 11.7a). In other instances, they are difficult to recognize because they are present in very low numbers; in this case, acid-fast stain (Ziehl–Neelsen or Kinyoun) may be helpful in recognition of bacteria (Figure 11.7b).

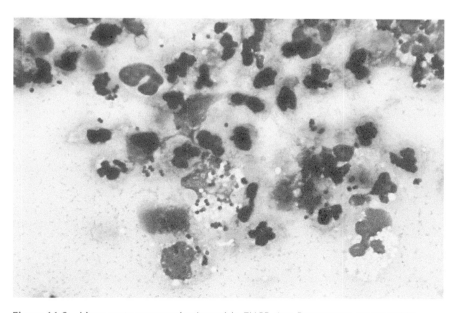

Figure 11.2 Liver, acute suppurative hepatitis, FNCS, dog. Degenerate neutrophilic granulocytes that show phagocytosis of coccoid bacteria (MGG, 100×).

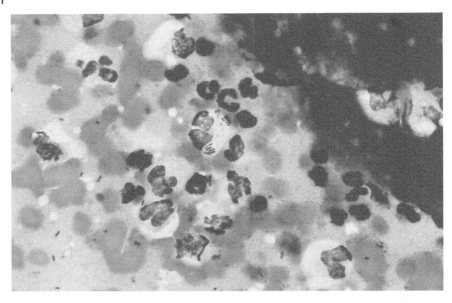

Figure 11.3   Liver, acute suppurative hepatitis, FNCS, dog. Degenerate neutrophilic granulocytes that show phagocytosis of rod-shaped bacteria (MGG, 100×).

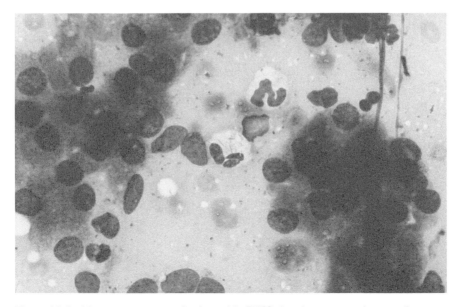

Figure 11.4   Liver, acute suppurative hepatitis, FNCS, dog. Among two clusters of hepatocytes, a degenerate neutrophilic granulocyte that demonstrates phagocytosis of elongated, filamentous bacteria (MGG, 100×).

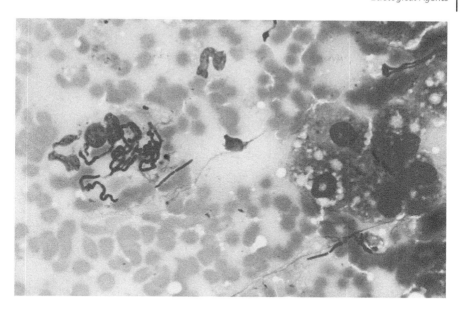

Figure 11.5 Liver, acute suppurative hepatitis, FNCS, dog. On the left, a small group of denegerate neutrophilic granulocytes that surrounds filamentous bacteria. Notice the casts of biliary material among the hepatocytes (MGG, 100×).

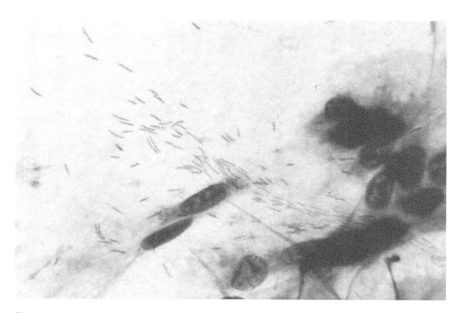

Figure 11.6 Normal gastric mucosa, squash prep, dog. *Helicobacter* spp. in a sample from gastric mucosa (100×).

(a)

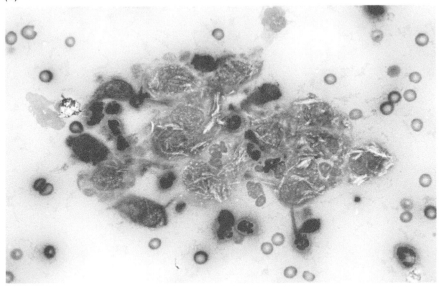

(b)

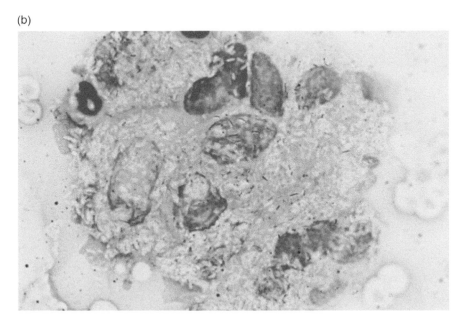

Figure 11.7   (a) Liver, subacute hepatitis, FNCS, dog. A high number of negative-staining rods, representing *Mycobacterium* spp. agents, within the cytoplasm of macrophages (MGG, 100×). (b) Liver, subacute hepatitis, FNCS, dog. Acid-fast stain is positive for the rod-shaped mycobacteria (Ziehl–Neelsen, 100×).

11.3 Protozoa

Leishmania spp. are causative agents of chronic hepatitis, typically characterized by granulomas in the fibrous support of portal tracts. Cytologically (personal observations) and histologically [12], well-preserved neutrophils and macrophages containing amastigotes occur in association with hepatocytes (Figure 11.8). The amastigotes are ovoid, 1.5–2×2.5–5 µm in diameter, with pale blue cytoplasm that contains an eccentrically located small ovoid nucleus; perpendicular to the nucleus, a single kinetoplast, bar-shaped and deep blue, is present. Other protozoal agents responsible for hepatic inflammation include *Toxoplasma* spp., represented by tachyzoites or merozoites, ovoid to banana-shaped, 1–7 µm in length, with pale blue cytoplasm and an eccentrically located, small round to ovoid nucleus; tachyzoites or merozoites can be observed clustered or individualized, intracellular or extracellular (Figure 11.9) [13]. *Sarcocystis canis* in dogs [14] is morphologically very similar to *Toxoplasma* spp. and others apicomplexean protozoans, such as *Neospora* spp., and serology or molecular diagnosis is often necessary for a final diagnosis. *Cytauxzoon felis* in cats [13] is represented by numerous small, round to comma-shaped purple merozoites, 1–2 µm in diameter, that fill the cytoplasm of macrophages, with an eccentrically located nucleus with a prominent nucleolus.

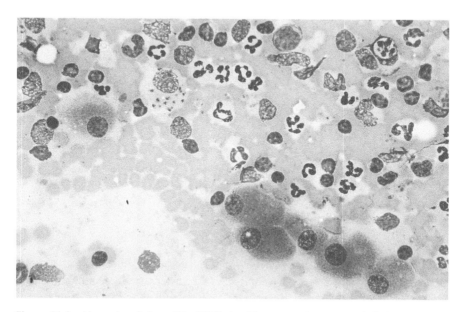

Figure 11.8   Liver, chronic hepatitis, FNCS, dog. The macrophage at top left demonstrates phagocytosis of amastigotes of *Leishmania* spp.; notice the normal hepatocytes on the bottom and many other inflammatory cells (MGG, 40×).

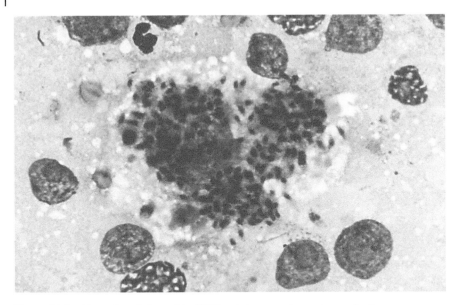

Figure 11.9   Liver, chronic hepatitis, FNCS, cat. A macrophage demonstrating phagocytosis of many tachyzoites of *Toxoplasma* spp. (MGG, 100×).

11.4   Fungi

Fungal infections of the hepatic parenchyma are extremely rare. Fungi are generally represented by elongated and septate hyphae with a basophilic cytoplasm and a thin, achromatic wall (Figure 11.10); fungal spores are round, 2–5 μm in diameter, with deep blue cytoplasm and a thin, clear wall. Fungal agents are generally surrounded by macrophages and sometimes by neutrophilic granulocytes. A case of a dog with fungal hepatitis and concurrent cobalamin deficiency has been described [15]. Cases of disseminated fungal infection with liver involvement have also been described [16].

11.5   Parasites

An infection of the trematode *Heterobilharzia americana*, determined by observation of ovoid to round basophilic thin-walled eggshell fragments and rare ciliated miracidia, has been described in a dog [17] (Figure 11.11). Eggs of *Amphimerus*

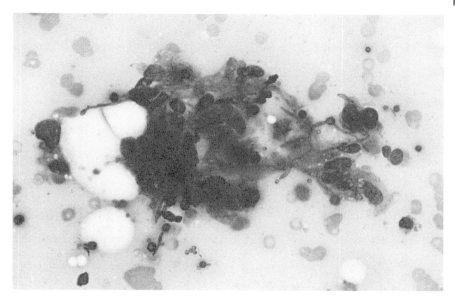

Figure 11.10   Liver, fungal hepatitis, FNCS, dog. A nest of branched fungal hyphae, surrounded by macrophages (MGG, 40×).

pseudofelineus [18] can be observed by fecal sedimentation, are opercolated and measure approximately 34–50 × 20–35 µm. *Platynosomum fastosum* [19] is a trematode that infects the feline liver, bile ducts, and gallbladder and is commonly found in tropical and subtropical regions, including the Caribbean islands, Central and South America, Asia, Australia, southern United States, and Hawaii; eggs, measuring 35.9 × 26.9 µm with a visible internal miracidium, may be present in bile. *Mesocestoides* spp. have been identified via fine needle aspiration of canine liver and mesenteric lymph nodes, without evidence of parasites in peritoneal fluid samples [20]. Cytology samples may contain large (200–400 × 500–2000 µm), oval to elongated, worm-like, deeply basophilic, granular structures consistent with cestode larvae and larval fragments, consistent with tetrathyridia; the larvae may contain numerous 1–2 µm, deeply basophilic, granular structures along with fewer numbers of larger (approximately 15 µm) clear to slightly yellow, refractile structures consistent with calcareous corpuscles [20].

In dogs affected by *Dirofilaria* spp., elongated larvae may be present among the hepatocytes (Figure 11.12): this finding, although suggesting a filariasis, should be interpreted as an incidental finding of larvae from blood contamination.

(a)

(b)

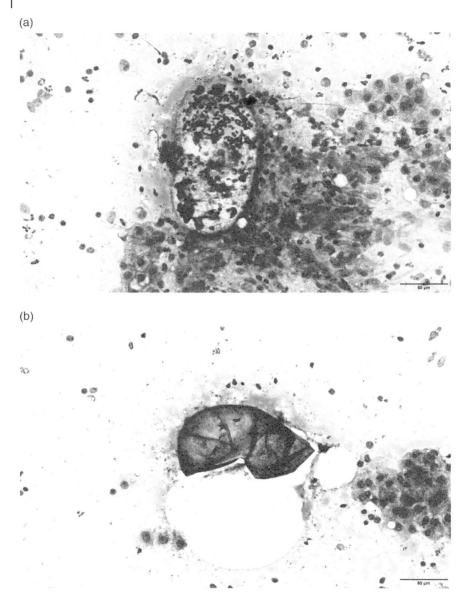

Figure 11.11 (a) Liver, parasitic hepatitis, FNCS, dog. A eggshell of *Heterobilharzia americana*, partially collapsed; compare the dimension of the egg with the hepatocytes on the background and on the right (MGG, 20×). (b) Liver, parasitic hepatitis, FNCS, dog. A miracidium of *H. americana* with internal nuclear structures; compare the dimension with the hepatocytes on the background (MGG, 20×). *Source:* Courtesy of Dr Shannon Dehghanpir.

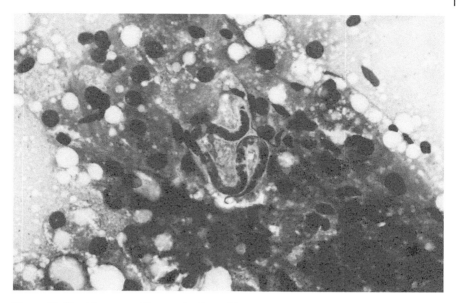

Figure 11.12 Liver, aspecific reactive hepatitis, FNCS, dog. A microfilaria of *Dirofilaria immitis* infiltrates a cluster of hepatocytes (MGG, 100×).

11.6 Key Points

- Etiological agents are much easier to identify with cytological examination than with histology.
- Viral diseases are difficult to observe and, although present, morphological evidence is an inconstant finding.
- When massive inflammation is present, mostly neutrophilic, always search carefully for bacteria.

References

1 Forrester, S.D., Rogers, K.S., and Relford, R.L. (1992). Cholangiohepatitis in a dog. *J. Am. Vet. Med. Assoc.* 200 (11): 1704–1706.

2 Kolios, G., Valatas, V., and Kouroumalis, E. (2006). Role of Kupffer cells in the pathogenesis of liver disease. *World J. Gastroenterol.* 12 (46): 7413–7420.

3 Meyer, D.K. (2016). *The Liver, Canine and Feline Cytology – A Color Atlas and Interpretation Guide*, 3e, 259–283. St Louis, MO: Elsevier.

4 Burr, P.D., Campbell, M.E., Nicolson, L., and Onions, D.E. (1996). Detection of canine herpesvirus 1 in a wide range of tissues using the polymerase chain reaction. *Vet. Microbiol.* 53 (3–4): 227–237.

5 Li, L., Pesavento, P.A., Leutenegger, C.M. et al. (2013). A novel bocavirus in canine liver. *Virol. J.* 13 (10): 54.

6 Li, L., McGraw, S., Zhu, K. et al. (2013). Circovirus in tissues of dogs with vasculitis and hemorrhage. *Emerg. Infect. Dis.* 19 (4): 534–541.

7 Wagner, K.A., Hartmann, F.A., and Trepanier, L.A. (2007). Bacterial culture results from liver, gallbladder, or bile in 248 dogs and cats evaluated for hepatobiliary disease: 1998–2003. *J. Vet. Intern. Med.* 21: 417–424.

8 Bishop, L., Strandberg, J.D., Adams, R.J. et al. (1979). Chronic active hepatitis in dogs associated with leptospires. *Am. J. Vet. Res.* 40: 839–844.

9 Fox, J.G., Drolet, R., Higgins, R. et al. (1996). *Helicobacter canis* isolated from a dog liver with multifocal necrotizing hepatitis. *J. Clin. Microbiol.* 34: 2479–2482.

10 Takemura, L.S., Marcasso, R.A., Lorenzetti, E. et al. (2019). Helicobacter infection in the hepatobiliary system and hepatic lesions: a possible association in dogs. *Braz. J. Microbiol.* 50 (1): 297–305.

11 Turinelli, V., Ledieu, D., Guilbaud, L. et al. (2004). Mycobacterium tuberculosis infection in a dog from Africa. *Vet. Clin. Pathol.* 33: 177–181.

12 Rallis, T., Day, M.J., Saridomichelakis, M.N. et al. (2005). Chronic hepatitis associated with canine leishmaniosis (*Leishmania infantum*): a clinicopathological study of 26 cases. *J. Comp. Pathol.* 132: 145–152.

13 Peters, L.M. and Meyer, D.J. (2023). Hepatobiliary system. In: *Canine and Feline Cytopathology*, 4e (ed. R.E. Raskin, D.J. Meyer, and K.M. Boes), 339–376. St Louis, MO: Elsevier.

14 Allison, R., Williams, P., Lansdowne, J. et al. (2006). Fatal hepatic sarcocystosis in a puppy with eosinophilia and eosinophilic peritoneal effusion. *Vet. Clin. Pathol.* 35 (3): 353–357.

15 Kook, P.H., Drögemüller, M., Leeb, T. et al. (2015). Hepatic fungal infection in a young beagle with unrecognised hereditary cobalamin deficiency (Imerslund-Gräsbeck syndrome). *J. Small Anim. Pract.* 56: 138–141.

16 Headley, S.A., de Mello Zanim Michelazzo, M., Elias, B. et al. (2019). Disseminated melanized fungal infection due to Cladosporium halotolerans in a dog coinfected with canine adenovirus-1 and canine parvovirus-2. *Braz. J. Microbiol.* 50 (3): 859–870.

17 Le Donne, V., McGovern, D.A., Fletcher, J.M. et al. (2016). Cytologic diagnosis of *Heterobilharzia americana* infection in a liver aspirate from a dog. *Vet. Pathol.* 53: 633–636.

18 Todd, K.S. Jr., Bergeland, M.E., and Hickman, G.R. (1975). *Amphimerus pseudofelineus* infection in a cat. *J. Am. Vet. Med. Assoc.* 166 (5): 458–459.

19 Stern, J.K., Walden, H.D.S., Marshall, K., and Sharkey, L. (2020). What is your diagnosis? Bile from a cat. *Vet. Clin. Pathol.* 49 (2): 354–355.

20 Patten, P.K., Rich, L.J., Zaks, K. et al. (2013). Cestode infection in 2 dogs: cytologic findings in liver and a mesenteric lymph node. *Vet. Clin. Pathol.* 42: 103–108.

12

Neoplastic Lesions of the Hepatic Parenchyma

While cytology may be considered too uncertain and inconclusive to diagnose most hepatic diseases, it redeems itself when it comes to recognizing the nature of almost all liver neoplasms. Ultrasound is an extremely reliable diagnostic tool to identify the presence of nodular lesions of the hepatic parenchyma [1], but its ability to establish the origin and nature of the neoplasm with certainty is limited. A fairly recent study demonstrated a low statistical correlation between the ultrasonographic findings of numerous pathological conditions affecting the hepatic parenchyma and the final histological diagnosis [2]. In another study [3], ultrasonographic discrimination between focal liver lesions of a benign and malignant nature identified the size of the lesion and the presence of effusion as the only two variables correlated with malignancy. The use of contrast-enhanced ultrasound (CEUS) has allowed progress in establishing the malignant nature of hepatocellular proliferation [4, 5], but in many cases, direct analysis of neoplastic cell morphology is necessary to formulate a definitive diagnosis. Therefore, cytological examination performed by fine needle sampling of the nodular parenchyma is probably the safest, most effective, and least invasive method to simultaneously discriminate neoplastic lesions [6] and, above all, to recognize the presence of malignancy criteria.

As ever, I need to underline how essential it is to compare the results of the cytological examination with the clinical and anamnestic findings, as the number and size of the lesions, the rate of progression, the evidence of primary lesions on other organs or lymph node metastases or on extrahepatic splancnic parenchyma are essential criteria to improve the diagnosis. Especially in uncertain cases, knowing the possible speed and evolution of the onset of the nodular lesion, establishing the presence in other organs of primary lesions that could metastasize to the liver or ascertaining whether the lesions are solid or cystic can contribute to producing a definitive diagnosis.

Canine and Feline Liver Cytology, First Edition. Carlo Masserdotti.
© 2024 John Wiley & Sons, Inc. Published 2024 by John Wiley & Sons, Inc.

When producing a morphological diagnosis, in addition to the need to have all the clinical, anamnestic, and ultrasound data, I believe it is important to briefly discuss one of the most underestimated technical aspects concerning the collection procedure. The presence of one or more nodular lesions of the parenchyma may initially induce the clinician to suspect a malignant neoplastic disease; the comparison between a sample from a nodular lesion and one from the nonnodular parenchyma should be used as preliminary evaluation, since similarity or diversity among the cells is a useful morphological feature in diagnosis. For example, cytological samples from nodular hyperplasia, one of the most common nodular lesions, frequently represented by multifocal lesions, consist of microscopically normal-looking hepatocytes often affected by reversible nonspecific damage, but whose characteristics do not differ consistently from nonnodular hepatic parenchyma samples. On the other hand, the difference between cells from a cholangiocarcinoma and from the surrounding parenchyma is strong enough to warrant a diagnosis of nonhepatocellular epithelial and malignant neoplasia. For this reason, my advice is to always acquire several samples simultaneously (both from the nodular lesion and the extranodular parenchyma), so as to be able to carry out an effective morphological comparison between the cells and, subsequently, recognize any differences.

In addition to the discussion below, the morphological similarity alone is sufficient to predict the proliferation of benign hepatocytes. Moreover, it must be remembered that in some instances, necrosis may be the largest part of a neoplasm and consequently the presence of necrotic debris sampled from a nodular lesion should always prompt suspicion of a tumor, to be further evaluated.

12.1 Epithelial Neoplasia

12.1.1 Nodular Hyperplasia

Cytomorphology: exfoliation of hepatocytes with round or polygonal cytoplasm, mostly normal in appearance, frequently affected by reversible nonspecific damage (Figures 12.1 and 12.2), which may be represented by accumulation of water, glycogen, or lipids; nucleus is round, sometimes double, with compact chromatin and nucleolate; hepatocytes aggregate in variably cohesive, bi- or three-dimensional sheets, sometimes with trabecular appearance (Figures 12.3 and 12.4); possible to observe a variable, generally mild degree of fibrosis (Figure 12.5); possible association with rare inflammatory elements.

This disorder, which is very common in elderly dogs and rare in cats, differs from regenerative nodules that arise in response to chronic damage of the hepatic parenchyma as a component of cirrhosis, on the basis of clinical, ultrasonographic

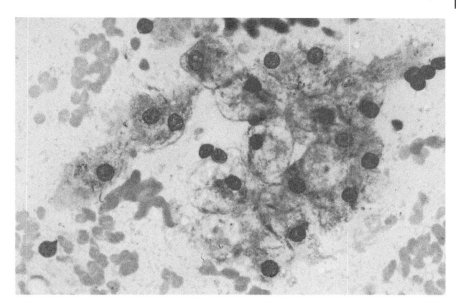

Figure 12.1 Liver, nodular hyperplasia, FNCS, dog. Note the achromatic, indistinct material accumulated within the cytoplasm and the absence of atypia (MGG, 100×).

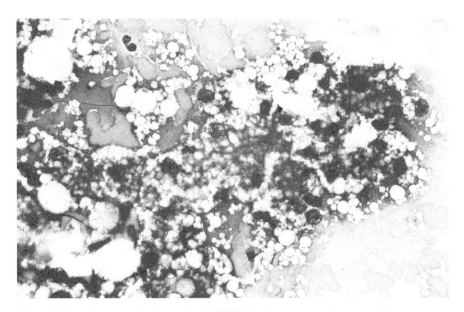

Figure 12.2 Liver, nodular hyperplasia, FNCS, dog. Hepatocytes from a nodular hyperplasia; cytoplasm may be filled with lipid globules; note the absence of atypia (MGG, 100×).

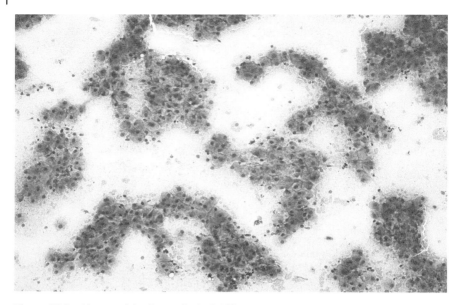

Figure 12.3   Liver, nodular hyperplasia, FNCS, dog. In nodular hyperplasia, hepatocytes may appear in branched, mostly cohesive trabeculae; note that hepatocytes are indistinguishable from nonnodular cells (MGG, 20×).

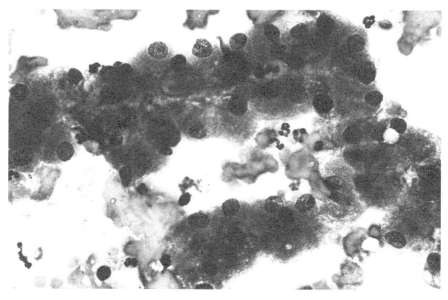

Figure 12.4   Liver, nodular hyperplasia, FNCS, dog. Although aspecific, rarely observed and not useful as a diagnostic feature, hepatocytes may arrange in bicellular trabeculae (MGG, 100×).

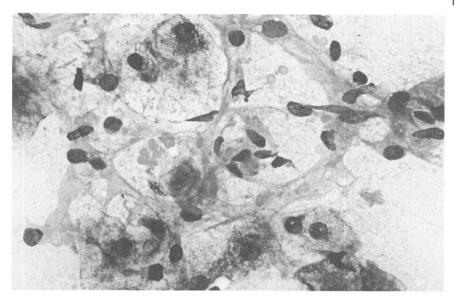

Figure 12.5   Liver, nodular hyperplasia, FNCS, dog. Among the hepatocytes from nodular hyperplasia, mild to moderate features of fibrosis may be evident (MGG, 100×).

data and of histological appearance, where fibrosis and necroinflammatory activity are not predominant features [7]. The precise causes are unknown, but it has been suggested that spontaneous nodular hyperplasia in the dog is stimulated by senile functional degradation of the parenchyma or may be induced artificially by feeding high-fat/low-protein diets [8]. No data suggest that nodular hyperplasia is a preneoplastic condition in dogs [7, 8]. Grossly, it can occur as single nodules (more frequently multiple), usually less than 3 cm in diameter, which may be fairly large and can bulge from the liver surface.

From a histological point of view, nodular hyperplasia generally consists of bi-tricellular trabeculae of hepatocytes that are either morphologically normal or affected by regenerative changes, such as water, glycogen, or lipid cytoplasmic accumulation, associated with dispersed portal spaces and centrilobular vessels [7]. The lesion lacks capsular containment and, in addition, it normally features a compact profile. In my opinion, its morphological characteristics are not sufficiently distinct to safely and conclusively exclude hepatocellular adenoma, particularly if diagnosis is done on a biopsy. This is mostly due to the fact that, in daily clinical practice, a clinician rarely performs an evaluation of the entire hepatic lobe containing the nodular lesion; therefore, it is not possible to analyze the edges of the lesion and their relationship with the surrounding hepatic tissue to determine the presence of a capsule or infiltrative behavior.

Cytologically, fine needle sampling of hyperplastic nodules generally provides hepatocytes that are either morphologically normal or affected by cytoplasmic accumulation of lipidic or glycogenic material; consequently, distinction from a healthy liver, or one that is affected by nonspecific degenerative changes, is difficult or impossible. For this reason, a comparison between nodular and nonnodular parenchyma may not show differences among hepatocytes.

12.1.2   Hepatocellular Adenoma

Cytomorphology: exfoliation of hepatocytes with round or polygonal cytoplasm, mostly normal in appearance, frequently affected by reversible nonspecific damage, which may be represented by cytoplasmic accumulation of water, glycogen, or lipids; nucleus is round, occasionally double, with compact chromatin and a single nucleolus; aggregation in variably cohesive, bi- or three-dimensional sheets (Figure 12.6); possible to observe a variable, generally mild degree of fibrosis (Figure 12.7); possible association with rare inflammatory elements.

My opinion is based on the current literature on the subject, but at the cost of being proved wrong or labeled as superficial, I shall say that recognizing and

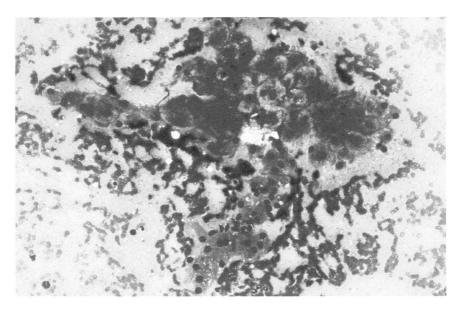

Figure 12.6   Liver, hepatocellular adenoma, FNCS, dog. A cluster of hepatocytes from an hepatocellular adenoma: cells are indistinguishable from nonneoplastic hepatocytes and from hepatocytes from nodular hyperplasia; note the arrangement in trabeculae (MGG, 40×).

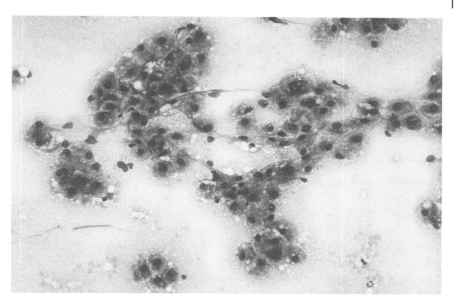

Figure 12.7 Liver, hepatocellular adenoma, FNCS, dog. A mild to moderate degree of fibrosis is sometimes present among benign hepatocytes from adenoma (MGG, 40×).

diagnosing a form of nodular hyperplasia and distinguishing it from a hepatocellular adenoma or even, in some cases, from a well-differentiated hepatocarcinoma is arbitrary and based on rather slender criteria. I do not believe I have ever diagnosed a hepatocellular adenoma with absolute certainty or established an obvious and clear difference from a form of nodular hyperplasia; histological features are represented by a roundish neoplasia, generally single, consisting of bi-tricellular trabeculae; portal tracts are rare and centrilobular vessels cannot be observed [7]. In practice, the only difference with nodular hyperplasia is a centrifugal growth that determines compression of the surrounding hepatic parenchyma, sometimes with thickening of fibrous tissue, but generally it lacks a capsule. Consequently, differentiation from a form of nodular hyperplasia, or even from a benign hepatocarcinoma, can be difficult (if not impossible), especially in samples obtained through biopsies.

In my opinion, the previously mentioned limits concerning the assessment of nodular hyperplasia can also be applied to this condition. The diagnosis is generally made on fragments of tissue obtained through biopsy, or on tissue that is insufficient to accurately assess the entire lesion edge and its relationship with the surrounding parenchyma. From a cytological point of view, diagnostic arbitrariness becomes even more marked; in fact, similarly to nodular hyperplasia, this condition is characterized by exfoliation of hepatocytes that are virtually indistinguishable from those considered normal and consequently, only comparison with clinical and ultrasound data may suggest a specific diagnosis.

Hepatocellular adenoma is a relatively rare condition, but the difficulty and sometimes arbitrariness in distinguishing it from nodular hyperplasia (and in some rare cases from well-differentiated hepatocarcinoma, as previously specified) suggest that the real diagnostic incidence is seriously warped by subjective diagnoses, based on incoherent and unreliable diagnostic criteria.

12.1.3   Hepatocellular Carcinoma

Cytomorphology: prevalence of hepatocyte aggregates with indistinct cytoplasm, affected by mild reversible and aspecific changes (Figures 12.8 and 12.9); anisokaryosis is generally mild, sometimes moderate, nuclei are round with granular to compact chromatin and a single nucleolus (Figure 12.10); in some rare cases, the nuclei may feature severe anisocytosis and anisokaryosis, with irregularly clumped chromatin and prominent nucleoli (Figures 12.11 and 12.12); frequently neoplastic hepatocytes are arranged in tridimensional clusters and show indistinct outline of the membrane, with loss of cell borders and disordered overlapping of the nuclei (Figure 12.13); a variable number of naked nuclei,

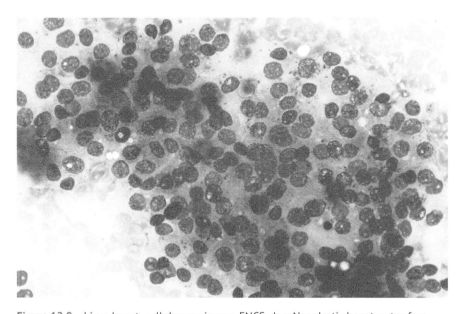

Figure 12.8   Liver, hepatocellular carcinoma, FNCS, dog. Neoplastic hepatocytes from well-differentiated hepatocellular carcinoma. The indistinct cytoplasms are sometimes filled with a very small amount of globular achromatic material and lipofuscin; note the overlapping of cells (MGG, 100×).

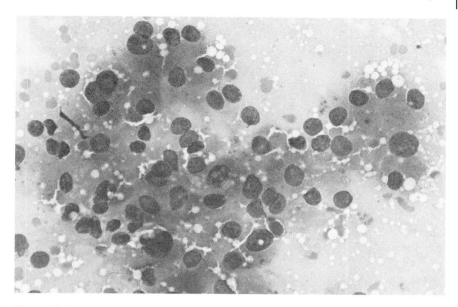

Figure 12.9 Liver, hepatocellular carcinoma, FNCS, dog. In some instances, globular achromatic material may be present in moderate amounts. Note the slight anisocytosis and overlapping of some cells (MGG, 100×).

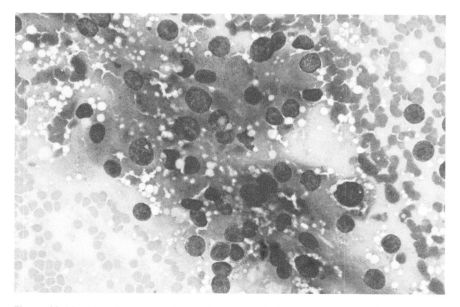

Figure 12.10 Liver, hepatocellular carcinoma, FNCS, dog. Neoplastic cells from a hepatocellular carcinoma; note the slight to moderate anisokaryosis, anisocytosis, and overlapping of cells (MGG, 100×).

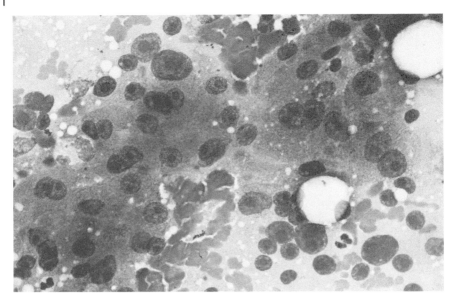

Figure 12.11   Liver, hepatocellular carcinoma, FNCS, dog. Anisokaryosis and anisocytosis are sometimes marked; note the presence of naked nuclei at bottom right (MGG, 100×).

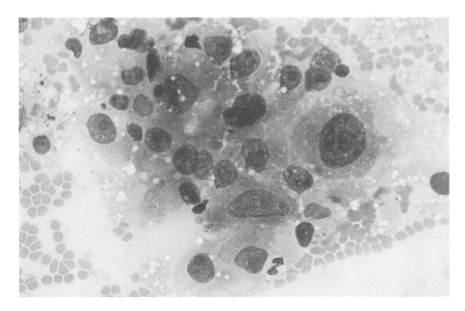

Figure 12.12   Liver, hepatocellular carcinoma, FNCS, dog. Although anisokaryosis and anisocytosis are marked, the neoplastic cells retain the reticulated, bluish cytoplasm that helps in recognition of a hepatocellular origin (MGG, 100×).

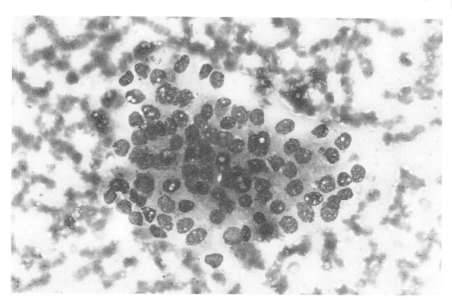

Figure 12.13   Liver, hepatocellular carcinoma, FNCS, dog. Neoplastic cells from hepatocarcinoma; note the indistinct cells borders, overlapping, and peripheral discohesion; anisokaryosis and anisocytosis are minimal (MGG, 100×).

sometimes high, crowd around hepatocyte aggregates (Figures 12.14 and 12.15); a microacinar or tubular arrangement of hepatocyte distribution can be observed (Figure 12.16).

Some unusual cytological characteristics of hepatocarcinoma include presence of bulky, weakly basophilic, dense, and refractile cytoplasmic inclusions with polygonal profile (Figure 12.17); perivascular arrangement may be a feature, where hepatocytes aggregate around a linear or branched capillary axis (Figures 12.18 and 12.19).

Hepatocellular carcinoma is generally represented by a nodular lesion or single mass. Histologically, it is characterized by the proliferation of elements with very variable morphology. In 1981, Patnaik described 11 morphological subtypes, each with particular morphological features [9]. Neoplastic cells range from well differentiated to markedly atypical, which can determine the formation of irregular trabeculae, supported by connective stroma and alternating with vascular lacunar spaces, in the absence of recognizable portal or centrolobular areas. Peripherally, it is possible to detect infiltration of the surrounding hepatic parenchyma, represented by digitation, trabeculae, nests, or small groups of neoplastic hepatocytes (Figure 12.20). This neoplasia may be observed in elderly or middle-aged dogs [7], while it is rare in the cat.

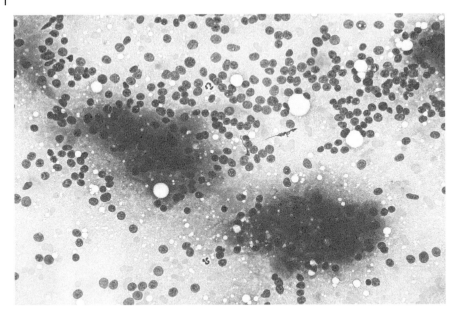

Figure 12.14 Liver, well-differentiated hepatocellular carcinoma, FNCS, dog. Many naked nuclei are crowded around two aggregates of neoplastic cells from a well-differentiated hepatocellular carcinoma (MGG, 40×).

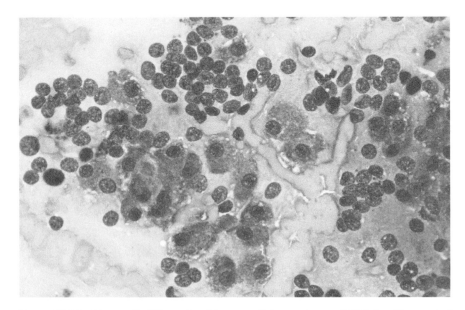

Figure 12.15 Liver, well-differentiated hepatocellular carcinoma, FNCS, dog. Many naked nuclei crowd around neoplastic epithelial cells; the cytoplasm and nucleus of this neoplastic cells appear almost normal in size and shape (MGG, 100×).

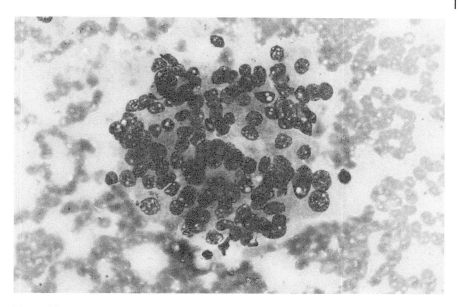

Figure 12.16 Liver, hepatocellular carcinoma, FNCS, dog. Irregularly distributed neoplastic cells, with a small amount of indistinct cytoplasm and round, overlapped nuclei; small microacinar arrangements are evident; note the small degree of anisocytosis and anisokaryosis (MGG, 100×).

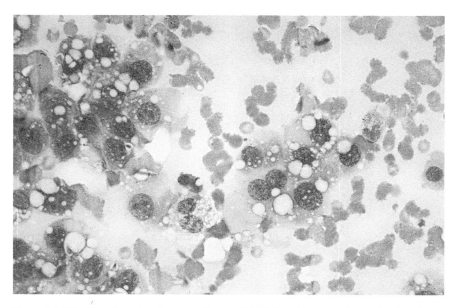

Figure 12.17 Liver, hepatocellular carcinoma, FNCS, dog. A large, polygonal, refractile, slightly basophilic body within the cytoplasm of the neoplastic cells in the center (MGG, 100×).

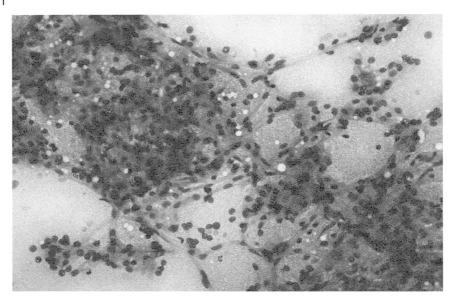

Figure 12.18 Liver, well-differentiated hepatocellular carcinoma, FNCS, dog. Aggregates of neoplastic hepatocytes crossed by branched capillaries (MGG, 40×).

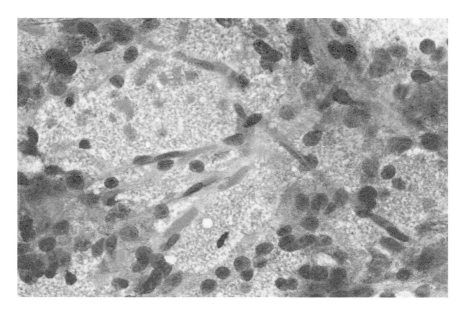

Figure 12.19 Liver, well-diferentiated hepatocellular carcinoma, FNCS, dog. Capillaries are recognizable as linear, sometimes branched structures, with spindle endotheliocytes and elongated nuclei. Note the red blood cells within the capillaries' lumina (MGG, 100×).

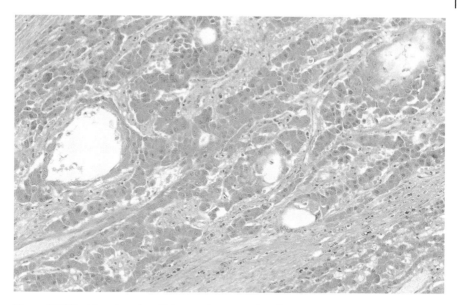

Figure 12.20   Liver, hepatocellular carcinoma, trabecular pattern, dog. Variably thick trabeculae infiltrate the stroma. Notice the low degree of atypia (HE, 40×).

I could provide a list of the usual clinical information found in oncology texts but in this case, I feel compelled to disagree, as I believe this is a lesion that generally manifests slow growth, with compression of the surrounding parenchyma and, in some more severe cases, may cause a superficial rupture with cavitary hemorrhage, rather than tumor spread. On the basis of previous reports, hepatocellular carcinoma may show a metastatic rate from 25% to 61% of cases [10]. Despite these data, I have always considered this form of neoplasm an oncological enigma; in fact, against all the morphological evidence that meets the criteria for malignancy, it is very unlikely to cause widespread infiltration, intrahepatic metastasis, the involvement of the lymph nodes or distant metastases, as commonly observed in other types of nonhepatocellular carcinoma. Furthermore, in those cases confirmed by cytological and histological diagnosis where the lesion has been radically removed, I have never observed any cases of recurrence or late metastasis.

In light of the above, I question the malignancy of this neoplasm, which is very aggressive in humans. Consequently, the diagnosis of hepatocellular carcinoma must be interpreted as the presence of morphological criteria fits with the description of published data, since this is not necessarily a life-threatening disease. Indeed, in my experience, dogs with hepatocellular carcinoma die more frequently from rupture of the neoplasm and hemorrhage than from metastases.

Cytological evaluation allows detection of sufficient diagnostic criteria to identify tangible differences from any other primary disease affecting the hepatic parenchyma. First, the disordered overlapping of neoplastic hepatocytes is a very useful criterion, although this aspect can be confused with the three-dimensionality of a normal liver cell aggregate. By "overlap," I mean a specific aspect of the neoplastic liver which is difficult to define: clusters of cells in which it is no longer possible to recognize the edges of the individual cells and the nuclei seem to coalesce into an amalgam of uniform cytoplasmic material. The crowding of naked nuclei at the periphery of the neoplastic aggregates is another criterion that must be interpreted correctly [11]. It is not represented by rare, random nuclei scattered on the background, which could come from the breakdown of cells weakened by nonspecific damage, but by numerous and variably aggregated groups of nuclei around clusters of neoplastic cells. I consider this morphological criterion a very useful marker of well-differentiated hepatocellular carcinoma [11]. The structure of the neoplastic cell is somehow weakened by the neoplastic transformation and, considering that on a histological basis there is no destruction of single cells, I believe the sampling and smearing procedures contribute significantly to the rupture of the cytoplasm and the consequent dispersal and aggregation of naked nuclei.

With the exception of microacinar or tubular formations, which in my opinion are extremely rare, I would like to discuss one of the many peculiar architectural aspects, namely perivascular distributions. This arrangement is represented by aggregates of neoplastic hepatocytes, possibly already affected by the criteria described above, which tend to organize around a linear or branched axis of endotheliocytes. This is a cytological aspect that should not be underestimated, as the vascular axis cannot detach from a nonneoplastic liver, first, because the actual vascular structures are surrounded by the portal or centrilobular connective tissue (and therefore cannot exfoliate), and second, because the sinusoids are not real vascular channels but consist of specific endotheliocytes that are fenestrated but lack basal membrane. In the neoplastic liver, the neoangiogenesis induced by the neoplasm may represent the origin of both the perivascular vessels and the cytological arrangement I have described. One of the subtypes of hepatocarcinoma described by Patnaik in 1981 is the so-called hepatocarcinoma with a peritheliomatous pattern, where the parenchyma is intersected by exuberant capillaries. Generally speaking, the vascular component that intersects the neoplastic aggregates is represented by a rare capillary axis, but I have seen some cases where the vascular network was exuberant, branched, and anastomosed.

In one hepatocarcinoma case, I detected weakly basophilic, diaphanous, reflective, irregularly polygonal cytoplasmic inclusions, which tended to deform the nucleus and the cytoplasmic profile [12]. The ultrastructural analysis identified these structures as accumulations of proteinaceous material of presumed plasma derivation. The cytologically observed inclusions could therefore correspond to the so-called "protein droplets," which are described in the WSAVA standard – believed to be proteinaceous accumulation consequent to shock, ischemia, or acute hepatocellular damage [13].

In addition to these hyaline bodies, a modest number of small eosinophilic cells have been described in hepatocarcinoma of the dog [11]. The finding is supported by observations of hepatocarcinoma in humans, where Mallory bodies [14], accumulations of alpha-1-antitrypsin [15], fibrinogen [16], and hyaline inclusions have been described [17, 18]. In very rare cases, bulky macronucleoli stand out both in the nucleus contained in neoplastic cells and in the bare nuclei that coalesce around the aggregates. In the description of the hepatocarcinoma subtypes by Patnaik [9], at least three types – cobblestone type, pleomorphic, and solid – are characterized by the presence of prominent macronucleoli.

In conclusion, I would like to point out that the neoplastic hepatocytes rarely express the characteristics of classic nuclear and cytoplasmic morphological atypia, such as those that may be observed in samples from carcinomas of other anatomical sites. However, also in those cases where marked atypia is detected – such as nuclear dysmetria, zollate chromatin or macronucleoli – the behavior of the neoplasm does not change much. After almost 30 years of studying liver cytology, I have still not come across a case featuring neoplastic hepatocytes metastatic to the lymph node or other splanchnic parenchyma so, despite the findings in human medicine, I am not convinced that hepatocarcinoma can be considered a true malignant neoplasm in dogs.

12.1.4 Cholangioma

Cytomorphology: the epithelial elements of biliary origin aggregate in two-dimensional (rarely three-dimensional) cohesive sheets and disperse on a proteinaceous, slightly bloody, and granular background (Figure 12.21), where normal hepatocytes – or those affected by mild changes of nonspecific damage – are rarely detected; epithelial cells show indistinct, roundish, or cuboidal cytoplasm, weakly basophilic, containing a round to ovoid nucleus, with granular or compact chromatin (Figure 12.22).

Cholangioma has the same characteristics as a generally single nodular or massive lesion of variable size, with a cystic or lacunar multilocular appearance in the cystadenoma variant, which is easily described with the aid of ultrasound examination [19]. These lacunar structures are filled with liquid, whose content is represented by the proteinaceous material observed on the background. From a histological point of view, cholangioma is a benign neoplasm deriving from the biliary structures, consisting of lacunar spaces filled with liquid proteinaceous material, delimited by monostratified epithelium of biliary origin, supported by stromal septa, with a generally centrifugal expansion that compresses the surrounding hepatic parenchyma [7] (Figure 12.23). As a direct consequence of the composition of the lesion (cystic spaces), exfoliation is generally poor and represented by rare biliary cells from the epithelial wall scattered on the background proteinaceous material.

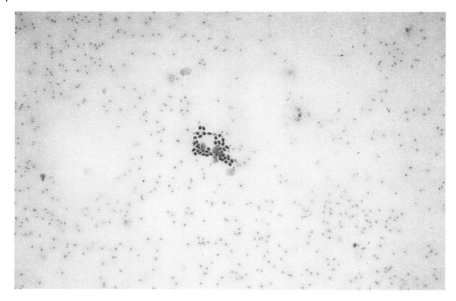

Figure 12.21 Liver, cholangioma, FNCS, cat. On a proteinaceous, slightly bloody background, there is a small aggregate of normal cholangiocytes, arranged in bidimensional sheets (MGG, 20×).

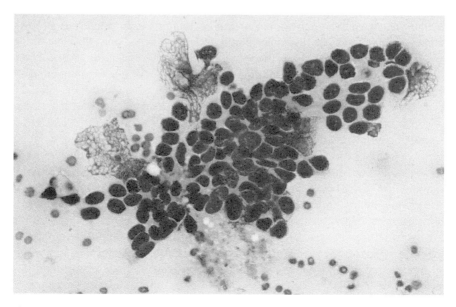

Figure 12.22 Liver, cholangioma, FNCS, cat. A sheet of benign cholangiocytes from a cholangioma; note the small, indistinct cytoplasm and the round to ovoid nuclei with compact to granular chromatin. Some cells, around the borders of the aggregate, seem to be disrupted (MGG, 100×).

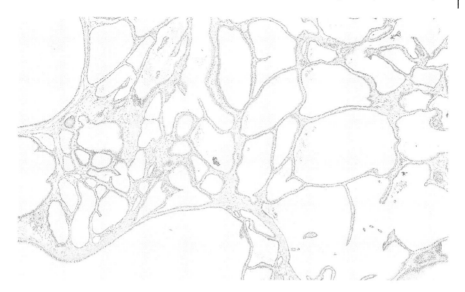

Figure 12.23 Liver, cholangioma, cat. Cystic structures lined with a single layer of well-differentiated biliary epithelium, supported by stroma (HE, 20×).

12.1.5 Cholangiocellular Carcinoma

Cytomorphology: epithelial elements with rounded, cuboidal, or indistinct, variably basophilic cytoplasm, sometimes filled with achromatic globules (Figure 12.24); nuclei are round to ovoid, with coarse to clumped chromatin and a single prominent nucleolus (Figure 12.25); anisokaryosis and anisocytosis are generally marked (Figure 12.26); the neoplastic elements are organized in sheets of variable size, with a dischoesive bi- or three-dimensional profile, with possible presence of microacinar structures (Figure 12.27), sometimes irregular rows, sometimes tubular formations (Figure 12.28); the neoplastic cells may be embedded in variable amounts of fibrillary, eosinophilic material (Figure 12.29). It is possible to observe associated groups of hepatocytes affected by nonspecific damage, together with morphological features of extracellular cholestasis (Figure 12.30), inflammatory elements, sometimes in high number, and debris, at times of seemingly necrotic origin, on the background (Figure 12.31).

Similarly to its benign version, cholangiocarcinoma derives from the cholangio-cytes that form the intrahepatic bile ducts; gross morphology is characterized by the presence of single nodules (more frequently multiple) with an umbilicated surface; a variant with cystic areas is called cholangiocellular cystadenocarcinoma [7]. Very frequently, at the time of diagnosis, the parenchyma is occupied by multiple coales-cent lesions, sometimes with widespread replacement of the organ. It is a very aggressive neoplasm that can develop metastases with a rate from 60% to 88% [10, 20]. Nevertheless, complete excision of localized cholangiocellular carcinoma,

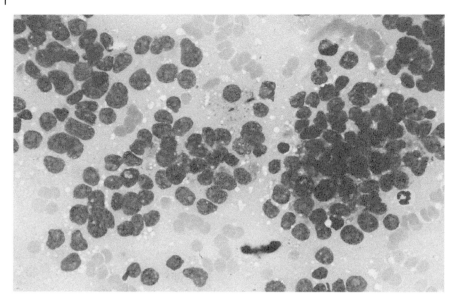

Figure 12.24 Liver, cholangiocellular carcinoma, FNCS, dog. Cells demonstrate indistinct, slightly blue cytoplasm, filled with a small amount of achromatic globules; chromatin is irregularly clumped; a single nucleolus is sometimes visible. Note the moderate degree of anisocytosis and anisokaryosis (MGG, 100×).

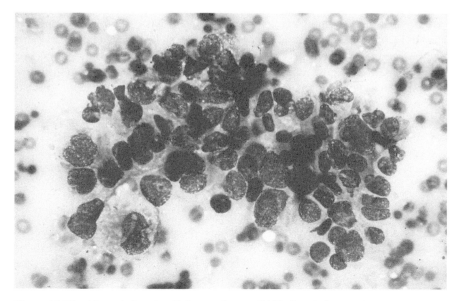

Figure 12.25 Liver, cholangiocellular carcinoma, FNCS, dog. A cluster of neoplastic cholangiocytes; the cytoplasm is indistinct and slightly blue; there is marked anisocytosis and anisokaryosis; chromatin is irregularly clumped and rare prominent nucleoli are evident. Note the focal arrangement in rows (MGG, 100×).

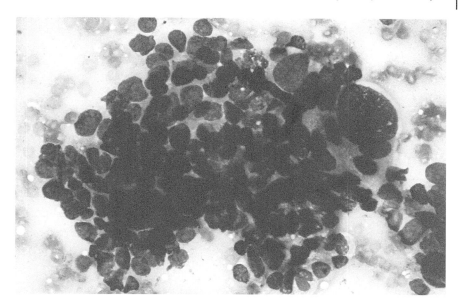

Figure 12.26   Liver, cholangiocellular carcinoma, FNCS, dog. In cholangiocellular carcinoma, anisokaryosis and anisocytosis are sometimes severe (MGG, 100×).

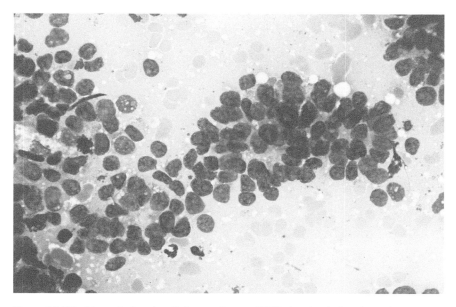

Figure 12.27   Liver, cholangiocellular carcinoma, FNCS, dog. In cholangiocarcinoma, a microacinar arrangement should be quite evident and represented by distribution of the cells around a small central area (MGG, 100×).

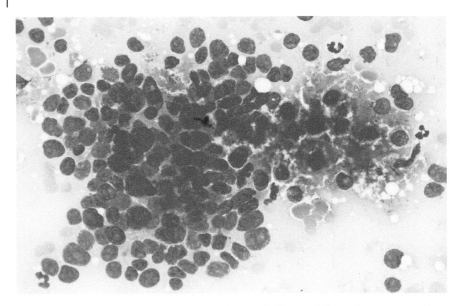

Figure 12.28 Liver, cholangiocellular carcinoma, FNCS, dog. Cells are here arranged in a discohesive cluster; note the presence of rows and tubular arrangements. On the right, for comparison, there is a small aggregate of hepatocytes (MGG, 100×).

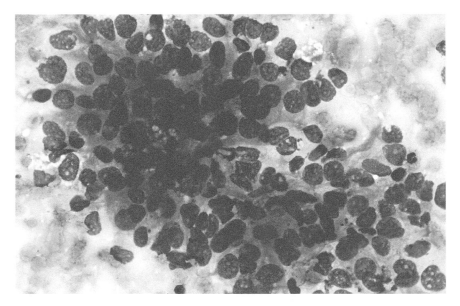

Figure 12.29 Liver, cholangiocellular carcinoma, FNCS, dog. Neoplastic cells may be embedded in fibrillary eosinophilic material, probably of stromal origin (MGG, 100×).

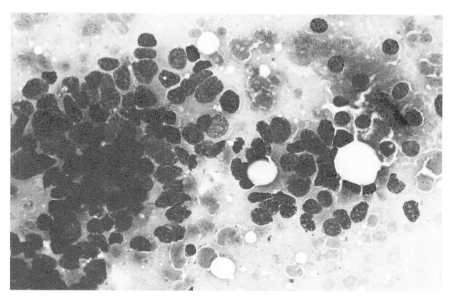

Figure 12.30 Liver, cholangiocellular carcinoma, FNCS, dog. On the right, there is a linear cast of biliary material among hepatic cells; the other cells from a cholangiocellular carcinoma are present in microacinar arrangements (MGG, 100×).

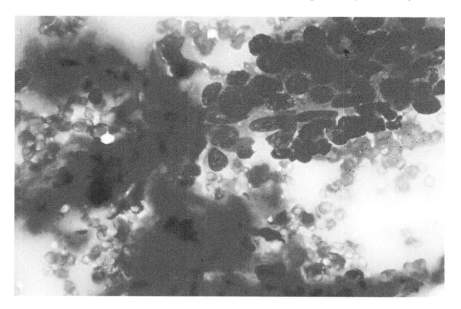

Figure 12.31 Liver, cholangiocellular carcinoma, FNCS, dog. A large amount of necrotic material surrounding a sheet of neoplastic cells from a cholangiocellular carcinoma (MGG, 100×).

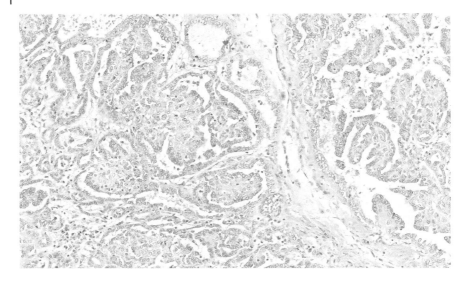

Figure 12.32 Liver, cholangiocarcinoma, dog. Tubular and acinar structures, lined by multiple rows of neoplastic cells, with occasional papillary projection (HE, 40×).

together with appropriate postsurgical therapy, has been proven to be curative in 66% of cases, although an early diagnosis is necessary for a favorable outcome [21].

Histologically, the neoplasm is characterized by the proliferation of tubular and acinar structures (Figure 12.32), frequently containing mucinous, periodic acid-Schiff (PAS)-positive material. These structures are dispersed in abundant stroma, with diffuse infiltration of the surrounding parenchyma; an abundant deposition of collagen, termed "scirrhous response," is relatively common. The cytomorphological features of cholangiocarcinoma are not necessarily specific; in fact, they could even be similar to metastases of extrahepatic neoplasms of epithelial origin, such as carcinomas of intestinal, pancreatic, renal, or prostate origin.

Personally, when I observe malignant epithelial neoplasms with the characteristics described above, I always advise the clinician to immediately ascertain the existence of any primary extrahepatic neoplasms through the use of imaging technology, as well as to investigate any anamnestic data that report previous extrahepatic neoplasms that have been removed but were never followed up by histological diagnosis. If the conditions necessary to hypothesize a primary extrahepatic epithelial neoplasm with liver metastasis do not occur, the final diagnosis is cholangiocarcinoma.

12.1.6   Other Nodular Lesions of Biliary Origin

It is important to remember that, in ultrasonographic investigations, some lesions of biliary derivation may resemble cysts with either zonal or nodular distribution. Indeed, there are known growth defects of biliary derivation, such as Caroli disease or the von Meyenburg complex, which feature expanded cystic structures surrounded by biliary cells. This is not the right place to discuss all biliary growth defects, or their embryological origins. I do not have direct experience of cytological evaluation involving lesions of this type, as they are very rare and my experience of them is limited; however, I firmly believe that if I had the luck to attempt a cytological examination of such a lesion, the microscopic features would not be so different from what I learned by investigating benign neoplastic biliary lesions, such as cholangioma.

In conclusion, if the sample features abundant exfoliation of cholangiocytes on a protein background, aside from cholangioma, it is advisable to report the potential presence of growth defects, and to proceed with further clinical and histological investigations.

12.1.7 Hepatic Carcinoid

Cytomorphology: roundish epithelial cells with a small amount of inconsistent, slightly basophilic, sometimes granular or reticulated cytoplasm, occasionally filled with very small achromatic globules, containing round or oval nuclei, with irregular or compact chromatin, occasionally nucleolated; anisokaryosis and anisocytosis are minimal (Figure 12.33). The cells tend to arrange in three-dimensional, discohesive

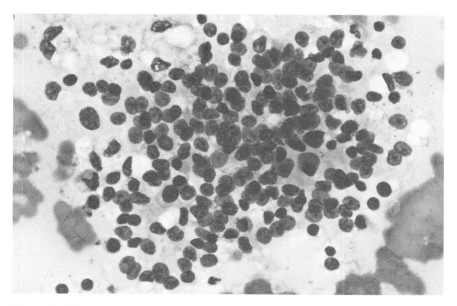

Figure 12.33   Liver, hepatic carcinoid, FNCS, dog. A sheet of epithelial neoplastic cells; notice the indistinct, finely granular, slightly basophilic cytoplasm and round nuclei, sometimes with a small nucleolus (MGG, 100×).

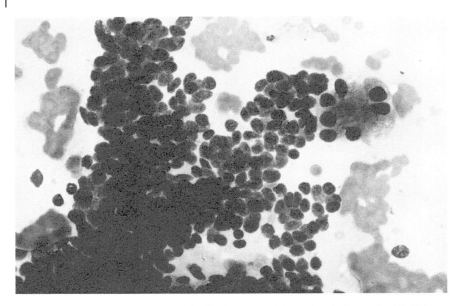

Figure 12.34 Liver, hepatic carcinoid, FNCS, dog. A tridimensional sheet of epithelial neoplastic cells; notice the slight disarrangement. On the right, there is a small group of hepatic cells for comparison (MGG, 100×).

aggregates (Figure 12.34); microacinar (Figure 12.35) and perivascular (Figure 12.36) arrangements may be observed in the epithelial sheets; the presence of naked nuclei that surround the epithelial aggregates is a frequent feature (Figure 12.37); possible association with groups of hepatocytes that are either normal or affected by nonspecific reversible changes; possible presence of debris and inflammatory elements.

The hepatic carcinoid presumably derives from neuroendocrine cells located in the epithelium of both intrahepatic and extrahepatic bile ducts; however, it may also derive from hepatic progenitor cells (also called oval cells), which in humans feature several of the morphological and immunohistochemical characteristics of the neuroendocrine elements [22]. Grossly, it may occur as a single mass or as multiple parenchymal nodules scattered throughout the liver, sometimes involving the large biliary ducts or the gallbladder, mostly in the cat [7]. The neoplastic tissue includes abundant tubular structures and rosette formations, distributed in vascularized branches of thin connective tissue (Figure 12.38), that sometimes is marked by fibrosis and mineralization. In the differential diagnosis, on the basis of the architectural presentation of the cells, cholangiocarcinoma or metastatic carcinoma of glandular origin must be excluded; carcinoid shows generally mild anisokaryosis and anisocytosis and, despite having the same arrangements, differs from cholangiocarcinoma as its microacinar structures are much more regular in shape, size, number, and distribution.

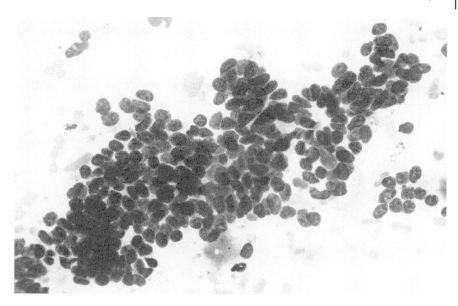

Figure 12.35 Liver, hepatic carcinoid, FNCS, dog. The neoplastic cells frequently show a microacinar arrangement (MGG, 100×).

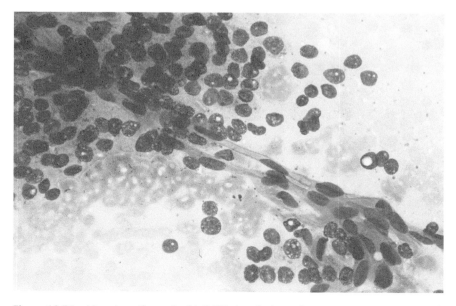

Figure 12.36 Liver, hepatic carcinoid, FNCS, dog. Perivascular arrangement, represented by a single vascular axis that crosses the sheet of neoplastic cells (MGG, 100×).

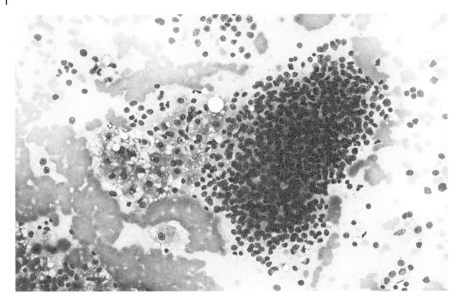

Figure 12.37 Liver, hepatic carcinoid, FNCS, dog. Many naked nuclei are crowded around the group of neoplastic cells or scattered on the background; note the presence of hepatic cells on the left side of the neoplastic sheet (MGG, 20×).

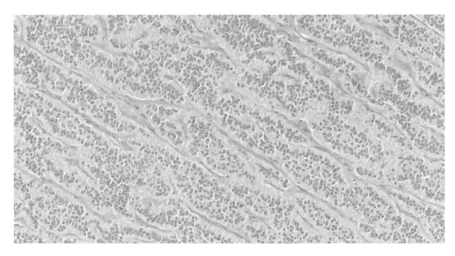

Figure 12.38 Liver, carcinoid, dog. Solid cords or ribbons of neoplastic cells separated by fine fibrovascular stroma (HE, 40×).

12.1.8 Hepatoblastoma

Cytomorphology: no personal experience.

Hepatoblastoma is an extremely rare neoplasm, described in the literature only in a elderly dog and in a cat [23, 24], that is believed to arise from hepatic progenitor cells. More hepatoblastomas have been reported in the equine [25] and ovine species [26]. The cytomorphological features of hepatoblastoma in a young horse have been described [27]; the cytological sample featured epithelial cells, smaller than hepatocytes, arranged in densely cellular cords, clusters, and occasional acinar-like arrangements. Individual epithelial cells have scant-to-medium blue cytoplasm and large but variably sized round nuclei; scattered mitotic figures were also noted. Hepatoblastoma is a benign neoplasm, although intra- and extrahepatic metastases have been reported in the horse [28].

12.2   Mesenchymal Neoplasia

12.2.1   Malignant Mesenchymal Neoplasms

Cytomorphology: a low to moderate number of spindle to tailed cells, with basophilic cytoplasm, containing a round or ovoid nucleus, with coarse to granular chromatin; nucleolus may be small or prominent; anisokaryosis and anisocytosis may be mild or marked; the spindle cells are organized in small bundles, sometimes embedded in pink, fibrillary strands of matrix and can be observed between aggregates of hepatocytes, normal, or affected by reversible aspecific changes (Figures 12.39 and 12.40); possible presence of inflammatory elements; in primary or metastatic hemangiosarcoma, neoplastic cells may arrange around vascular spaces, sometimes filled with erythrocytes (Figure 12.41).

Malignant mesenchymal neoplasms are generally metastases of a primary sarcoma, while the primary ones, in dog and cat, mostly represented by hemangiosarcoma, are extremely rare, with only a few reported osteosarcomas [29, 30], chondrosarcoma [31], leiomyosarcoma [32], peripheral nerve sheath tumor [33], liposarcoma [34], rhabdomyosarcoma [35], or fibrosarcoma [36]. Much more useful from a clinical point of view is establishing if the sarcoma is primary or metastatic; although primary liver sarcomas are very rare, without a complete clinical evaluation, mostly by imaging or, in some cases, a postmortem examination, a definitive diagnosis may be impossible. In addition to primary extrahepatic hemangiosarcoma, a gastrointestinal stromal tumor, that generally originates in the gastrointestinal wall and derives from the interstitial cells of Cajal, may metastasize to the liver, mesenteric lymph node, and omentum in 28% of dogs [37].

The cytological characteristics of mesenchymal tumors are rarely specific. In fact, although it is normally possible to recognize their mesenchymal features and to reach a diagnosis of sarcoma, it is almost impossible to observe specific

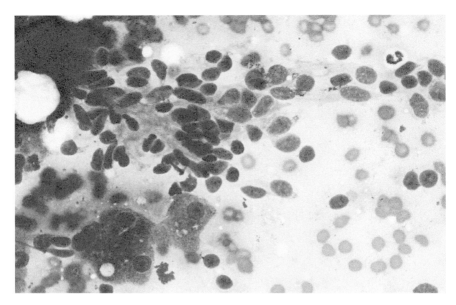

Figure 12.39 Liver, hepatic sarcoma, FNCS, dog. Spindle cells with elongated, tailed, or indistinct, slightly blue cytoplasm with ovoid nuclei; anisocytosis and anisokaryosis are moderate; note the presence of thin strands of eosinophilic material among the cells (MGG, 100×).

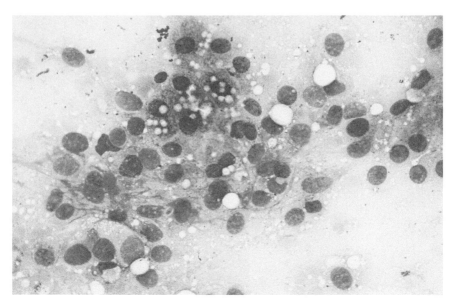

Figure 12.40 Liver, hepatic sarcoma, FNCS, dog. Spindle cells with elongated, tailed, slightly blue cytoplasm with ovoid nuclei; anisocytosis and anisokaryosis are severe; the cells are embedded in strands of eosinophilic, fibrillary material. Note the presence of hepatocytes at the top, for comparison (MGG, 100×).

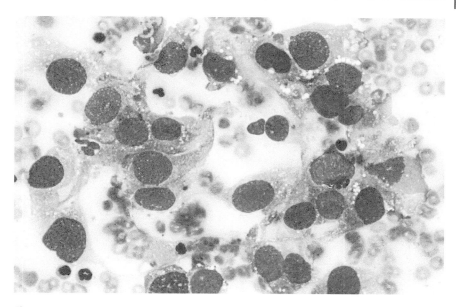

Figure 12.41 Liver, hemangiosarcoma, FNCS, dog. Spindle cells with elongated, tailed, or indistinct, slightly blue cytoplasm with ovoid nuclei; the cells arrange around irregular spaces filled with erythrocytes (MGG, 100×).

morphological features that allow prediction of the histotype of derivation. In many cases of mesenchymal neoplasia, immunohistochemistry on bioptic tissue is the only reliable procedure to correctly recognize the origin of the neoplasm; in some case, the morphological features of hemangiosarcoma, where malignant cells may arrange around luminal spaces (Figure 12.42), reminiscent of vascular channels, may help in diagnosis [38].

12.3 Hematopoietic Neoplasia

Hepatic involvement in hematopoietic neoplasia is readily recognized by a large number of round, discrete neoplastic cells among the hepatocytes. Their cytomorphological features are similar to those that can be detected in other organs or tissues and are mostly referable to the lymphoid, histiocytic, or mast cell cytotypes, as well as plasmocytoid and myeloid.

While the presence of neoplastic round cells in a cytological sample from liver generally indicates systemic or multiorgan involvement, a primary hepatic localization is also possible. Although a nodular presentation cannot be excluded, these types of neoplasm are macroscopically represented mostly by generalized enlargement of the liver with hyperechogenicity of the parenchyma. In histological sections, round cell tumors generally surround the portal tracts or the central veins

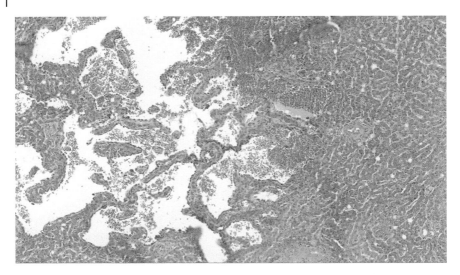

Figure 12.42   Liver, metastasis of hemangiosarcoma, dog. Endothelial cells line large, cystic, vascular spaces (HE, 40×).

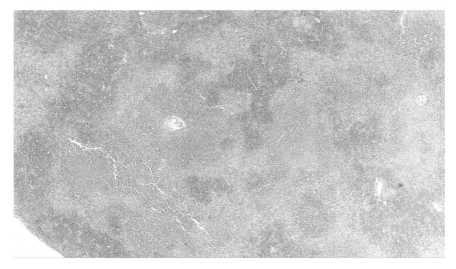

Figure 12.43   Liver, large cell lymphoma, dog. Neoplastic cells expand the borders of affected portal tracts and diffusely infiltrate the liver (HE, 20×).

or distribute along the sinusoids, although a nodular distribution is sometimes possible (Figure 12.43).

Generally, the cytological approach is sufficient to produce a diagnosis, but in some cases, to recognize the exact origin of neoplastic cells it may be necessary to perform an immunocytochemical or cytofluorimetric investigation, which can be carried out either on samples acquired by needle injection or on cytological smear. The cytological examination is in some cases inconclusive and polymerase chain reaction (PCR) for antigen receptor rearrangement (PARR) has become a common method to confirm or rule out a lymphoproliferative neoplasm.

12.3.1 Myelolipoma

Cytomorphology: presence, on bloody background, of hematopoietic cells that are easily recognizable when the myeloid and erythroid component is associated with megakaryocytes; presence of tridimensional clusters of mature adipocytes (Figure 12.44); presence of a variable number of normal hepatocytes.

Myelolipoma is a relatively rare neoplasm described only in domestic or wild cats [39, 40]. This is a generally multinodular neoplasm, varying in size from a few millimeters to several centimeters; the masses, localized in the hepatic parenchyma, are composed of hematopoietic cells distributed among lobules of normal and mature adipocytes; the edge of the mass is irregular, although sometimes outlined by a thin fibrous capsule. Recognition of hematopoietic cells together with mature adipocytes generally allows a definitive cytological diagnosis [41].

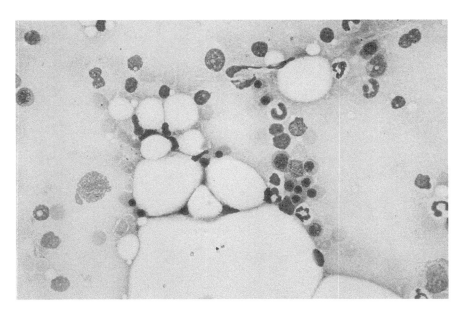

Figure 12.44 Liver, myelolipoma, FNCS, dog. Hematopoietic cells, mostly represented by erythroid and myeloid cells, are scattered among small groups of mature, normal adipocytes (MGG, 100×).

12.3.2 Large Cell Hepatic Lymphoma

Cytomorphology: large round cell with lymphoid appearance, generally greater than the diameter of two or three red blood cells (Figure 12.45); these cells have a variable amount of cytoplasm, gray to light blue in T-cell lineage (Figure 12.46), dark blue in B-cell lineage (Figure 12.47), sometimes with a clear polar halo. The cytoplasm may contain small achromatic globules; nuclei are large and roundish, occasionally with an irregularly outlined shape; chromatin is variably granular, coarse, or clumped; particularly in lymphoma of B-cell lineage, the nucleolus is large and prominent; atypical mytoses may be numerous, especially in lymphoma of T-cell lineage. The neoplastic cells may be numerous, effacing the hepatic cells; in many cases, neoplastic cells are scattered on the background or crowded around the hepatocyte clusters. Depending on the sample and preparation method, traumatized or ruptured neoplastic cells may appear as strands of nuclear material and cytoplasmic debris. Normal hepatocytes or hepatocytes with nonspecific, reversible damage, inflammatory cells, and debris may be detected; in some cases extracytoplasmic cholestasis is detectable (Figure 12.48).

Hepatic lymphoma may occur as a component of multicentric lymphoma, although primary disease has been described [42]. Although ultrasonography of the liver is specific but not sensitive in the detection of lymphomatous infiltration [43], in general liver involvement can be characterized by normal to slight reduction in hepatic echogenicity (compared with the renal cortex), anechoic or hypoechoic

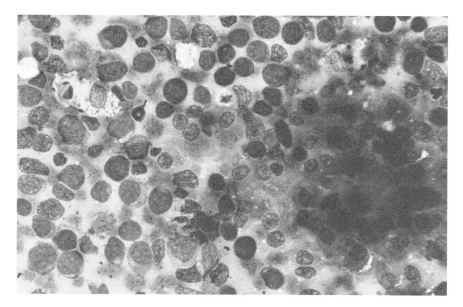

Figure 12.45 Liver, high-grade lymphoma, FNCS, dog. A single cluster of hepatocytes, on the right, is surrounded by a large number of large, discrete, round cells, with slightly basophilic cytoplasm, large round to ovoid nuclei and prominent nucleoli (MGG, 100×).

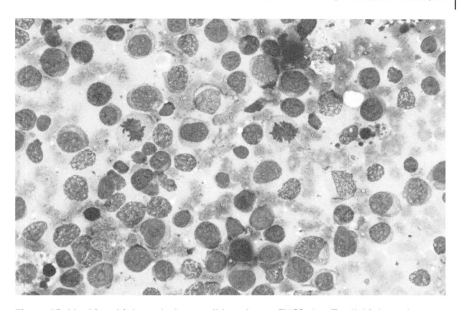

Figure 12.46   Liver, high-grade, large cell lymphoma, FNCS, dog. T-cell, high-grade lymphoma is frequently marked by large lymphoid cells with slightly basophilic cytoplasm and round to ovoid nucleus; chromatin is irregularly granular to clumped; nucleoli are rare and, when present, prominent; mitoses are numerous (MGG, 100×).

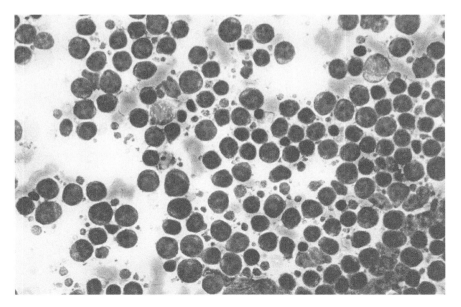

Figure 12.47   Liver, high-grade, large cell lymphoma, FNCS, dog. In B-cell, high-grade lymphoma, cells show deeply basophilic cytoplasm and round to ovoid nuclei with clumped chromatin; nucleoli are numerous, frequently multiple (MGG, 100×).

234 | *Canine and Feline Liver Cytology*

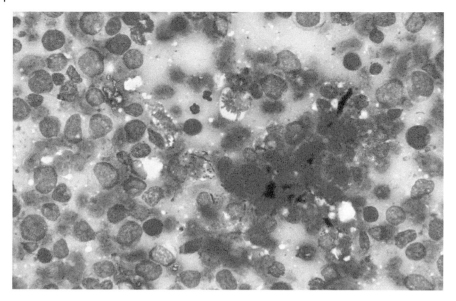

Figure 12.48   Liver, high-grade, large cell lymphoma, FNCS, dog. Cholestasis may be detectable among the hepatocytes, as a consequence of infiltration and obstruction of bile flow (MGG, 100×).

poorly marginated lesions or multiple round echodensities surrounded by areas of decreased echogenicity [44]. Consequently, since abnormal appearance of the liver on ultrasound examination is an indication that lymphoma is present in that organ, cytological evaluation should be used as the gold standard in confirming the diagnosis [45].

Although the morphological features (color of cytoplasm, presence of single or multiple macronucleolus) can help in recognition of a B- or T-cell lymphoma, establishing the phenotype of hepatic lymphoma with cytological evaluation can be difficult. When necessary for therapeutic choices or as a prognostic factor, exact recognition of the phenotype should be gained through cytofluorimetric or immunocytochemical methods. In this regard, when the cytological diagnosis is definitive for a diagnosis of hepatic lymphoma, I consider the use of biopsy superfluous; the only reason it may be performed is to obtain a fragment of tissue for immunohistochemical evaluation in cases where cytofluorimetry or immunocytochemistry is not enough to evaluate the phenotype.

12.3.3   Small Cell Lymphoma

Cytomorphology: small round cell with lymphoid appearance, with diameter generally comparable to that of an erythrocyte or slightly larger; these cells have a scanty amount of cytoplasm, generally gray to light blue; nuclei are small and

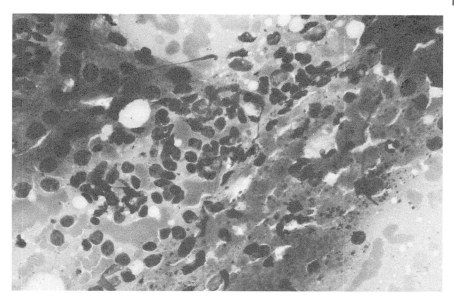

Figure 12.49   Liver, low-grade, small cell lymphoma, FNCS, cat. Small lymphocytes, with a thin rim of cytoplasm and round nucleus with compact chromatin, crowded in high numbers around a cluster of hepatocytes. No reliable features help in distinguishing small cell lymphoma from lymphocytic inflammation (MGG, 100×).

round; chromatin is generally granular to compact; the nucleolus is generally not visible; mitotic figures are generally absent. The neoplastic cells generally are scattered or distributed around the hepatocytes (Figure 12.49); normal hepatocytes or hepatocytes with nonspecific, reversible damage, inflammatory cells, and debris may be detected.

Small cell hepatic lymphoma mainly affects the cat and very rarely the dog. In cats, the diagnosis can be difficult as the presence of small lymphocytes is virtually indistinguishable from an inflammatory population as observed in lymphocytic cholangitis [46]; moreover, the presence of small, monomorphic lymphocytes could be consistent with infiltrative behavior of cells from chronic lymphocytic leukemia (CLL) in the liver. Definitively differentiating a lymphocytic cholangitis from a hepatic small cell lymphoma may also be difficult from a histological point of view and may require confirmation by immunohistochemical or clonality investigation [47].

It is not clear if this type of lymphoma develops as a primary neoplastic form, is associated with small cell intestinal lymphomas, or is the result of the transformation of severe and progressive forms of lymphocytic cholangiohepatitis. In this type of lymphoma, it is crucial to recognize the neoplastic transformation of the lymphocytes, which can be achieved directly on a cytological sample, through molecular-biological evaluations, or with the PARR method, with appropriate sensitivity and specificity to establish the presence of a tumor lymphoid clone.

12.3.4 Large Granular Lymphocyte (LGL) Lymphoma

Cytomorphology: intermediate to large-sized, round, lymphoid cells; these cells show light blue cytoplasm, filled with intensely eosinophilic, pink to magenta, multiple granules that are either dispersed or often crowded around the nucleus, at one pole of the cytoplasm (Figure 12.50); although in the cat these granules are easily recognizable, in the dog they may be thin and inconsistent (Figure 12.51); the nucleus is generally round, but may appear indented or with an irregularly shaped profile (Figure 12.52); chromatin may vary from compact to granular or clumped; nucleoli may be detected. The neoplastic cells are scattered, generally in high number on the background of the smear; when crowded around the hepatocyte sheets, they may clump and recognition of round shape may be difficult; in these cases, the presence of large granules is generally mandatory for diagnosis; possible presence of reversible, nonspecific hepatocellular damage and inflammatory elements (Figure 12.53); in some cases extracytoplasmic cholestasis is detectable.

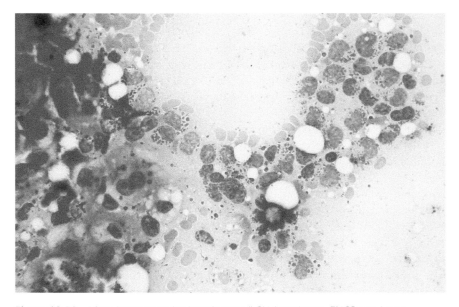

Figure 12.50   Liver, large granular lymphocyte (LGL) lymphoma, FNCS, cat. Large lymphoid cells contain prominent magenta cytoplasmic granules (MGG, 100×).

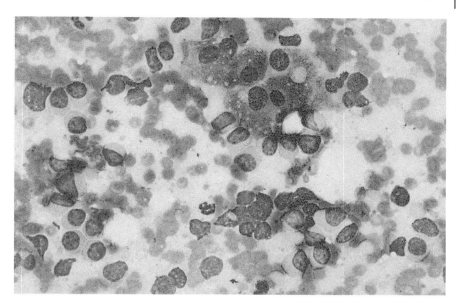

Figure 12.51 Liver, large granular lymphocyte (LGL) lymphoma, FNCS, dog. Neoplastic lymphoid cells contain multiple small magenta intracytoplasmic granules and nuclei with mature, clumped chromatin, and inapparent nucleoli (MGG, 100×).

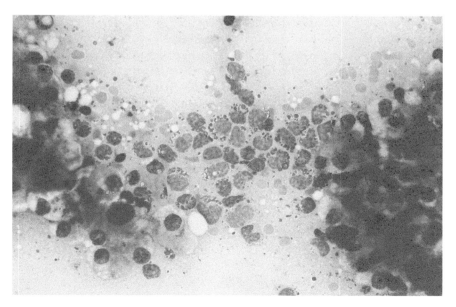

Figure 12.52 Liver, large granular lymphocyte (LGL) lymphoma, FNCS, cat. Nuclei show an irregular, sometimes folded profile and clumped chromatin (MGG, 100×).

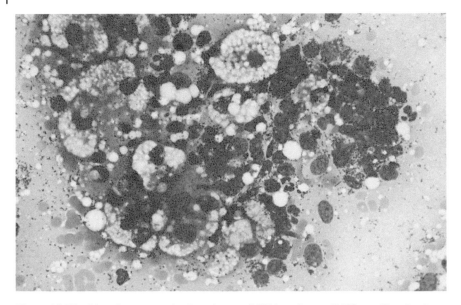

Figure 12.53 Liver, large granular lymphocyte (LGL) lymphoma, FNCS, cat. Neoplastic cells surround a group of hepatocytes, which contain small globules consistent with microvesicular steatosis (MGG, 100×).

Large granular lymphocyte (LGL) lymphoma is a subtype of lymphoma, easily recognizable by its peculiar appearance, based on the presence of cytoplasmic granules (so-called "azurophilic" granules because they stain with Azure A). An attempt to classify the morphological appearance of the neoplastic cells as mature (small size and uniform, fine granules), immature (large size and heterogeneous cytoplasmic granules) or immature (large size and coarse, up to 2 μm granules) has been reported [48]; however, the cytological appearance of LGLs did not appear to correlate with clinical outcome, which is characterized by aggressive biological behavior and poor prognosis.

LGL lymphoma is relatively common in felines, arises generally in the gastrointestinal tract and readily metastasizes to lymph nodes, spleen, and liver; bone marrow and peripheral blood involvement are frequent findings. The cytological diagnosis is generally definitive even if the lesion phenotype remains undetermined. Histological examination is not useful, not only because it does not add any supplementary information to the cytological diagnosis but mostly because cytoplasmic granules do not stain with standard hematoxylin-eosin stain.

Although phenotypic and molecular studies have assigned feline LGL lymphoma to either the cytotoxic T cell, CD3+, CD4+, CD8+ lineage or to a non-B non-T phenotype most consistent with NK cells, confirmation of a LGL lymphoma by immunohistochemistry is always difficult, if not impossible; for this reason, cytology is the most reliable method for a definitive diagnosis.

12.3.5 Epitheliotropic Lymphoma

Cytomorphology: small lymphoid round cells, with a diameter generally comparable to that of an erythrocyte or slightly larger; very thin rim of basophilic cytoplasm; nucleus is round, with compact chromatin; no nucleolus is detectable. The neoplastic lymphoid elements may manifest epitheliotropism, represented by their ability to enter the hepatocyte cytoplasm (Figures 12.54 and 12.55), which is affected by variable phenomena of nonspecific damage.

This is a very rare type of small cell lymphoma, representing a distinct biologic entity rather than a histologic variant of hepatosplenic T-cell lymphoma [49]. The epitheliotropic behavior is probably related to a phenomenon called "emperipolesis," defined as active penetration of one cell by another which remains intact [50]; this phenomenon differs from phagocytosis because the engulfed cell can exit from another cell without physiological or morphological consequences for either cell [51]. Other observations, by electron microscopy, revealed that the

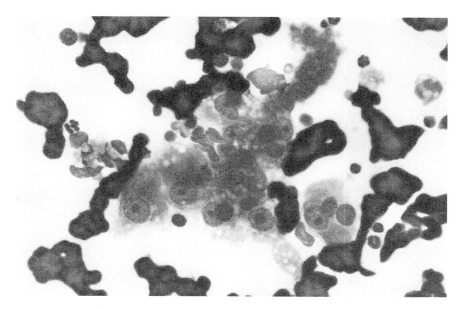

Figure 12.54 Liver, epitheliotropic lymphoma, FNCS, cat. Small lymphocytes enter the cytoplasm of the hepatocytes; some lymphocytes displace the nuclear outline (MGG, 100×).

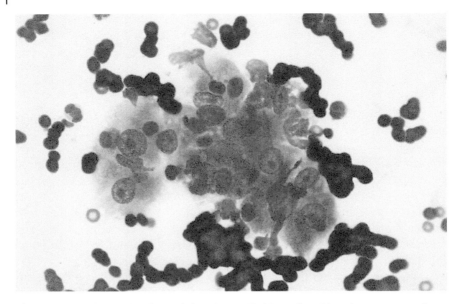

Figure 12.55 Liver, epitheliotropic lymphoma, FNCS, cat. Small lymphocytes enter the cytoplasm of the hepatocytes; some hepatocytes contain two lymphoid cells (MGG, 100×).

lymphocytes were not truly in the cytoplasm of hepatocytes and the appearance was due to invagination of the hepatocyte cell membrane [49]. Diagnosis requires careful and close evaluation, as it is not easy to fully detect the location of neoplastic lymphoid cells within the hepatocyte cytoplasm and clearly distinguish this from an overlap.

12.3.6 Other Types of Hepatic Lymphoma

Here we discuss some extremely rare types of liver lymphoma described in the literature. My experience of these is very limited but it is hoped that the readers of this book will acquire new knowledge about these rare types of neoplasm in order to provide useful information in future publications.

Sézary syndrome, a generalized epitheliotropic T-cell lymphoma, considered to be a variant of mycosis fungoides, accompanied by erythroderma, lymphadenopathy, and neoplastic T cells in peripheral blood, was described in the liver of a Boxer dog [52].

The so-called **hepatosplenic lymphoma** has a T-phenotype but a gamma-delta receptor; it infiltrates the liver, mostly in sinusoid and spleen. Dogs with hepatocytotropic T-cell lymphoma had different clinicopathological results, histological lesions, and immunophenotype which can be considered a separate clinical entity and not a subtype of hepatocytotropic lymphoma [53]. Neoplastic cells are intermediate to large, with large, round to irregularly outlined, sometimes indented nuclei. The cytological diagnostic key is the presence of erythrocytes inside the cytoplasm of the neoplastic lymphoid cells (Figure 12.56) and in the cytoplasm of associated macrophages, believed to be a form of erythrophagocytosis [53]. A hemophagocytic syndrome may be associated with hepatosplenic lymphoma [54].

B-cell lymphoma with Mott cell differentiation is considered to be a gastrointestinal lymphoma with involvement of mesenteric lymph nodes and liver, marked by the presence of lymphoblast and atypical Mott cells that contain many discrete, clear to pale blue cytoplasmic inclusions consistent with Russell bodies (Figure 12.57). The Mott cells, typically considered to be a plasma cell variant, are here represented by B-lineage neoplastic lymphoid cells, that accumulate large inclusions of nonsecreted immunoglobulins [55]. On the basis of these observations, this tumor most likely represents a variant of B-cell neoplasia with extensive Mott cell differentiation [56].

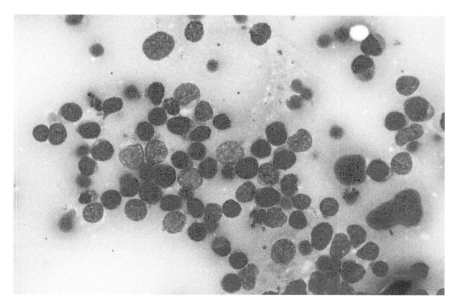

Figure 12.56   Liver, hepatosplenic lymphoma, FNCS, cat. The cytoplasm of neoplastic lymphoid cells frequently contains an erythrocyte (MGG, 100×).

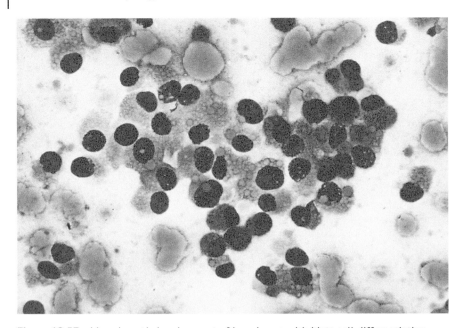

Figure 12.57   Liver, hepatic involvement of lymphoma with Mott cell differentiation, FNCS, dog. The cytoplasm of lymphoid neoplastic cells is filled with many achromatic, round globules, consistent with Russell bodies (MGG, 100×).

12.3.7   Malignant Histiocytic Neoplasms

Cytomorphology: exfoliation of large round, discrete elements, sometimes with tailed, spindled or stellate blue cytoplasm, sometimes containing small clear globules (Figure 12.58); the nucleus has a round, indented, sometimes irregularly folded profile, with coarse to clumped chromatin and prominent nucleolus; multiple nuclei are frequently observed (Figure 12.59). Cytophagocytosis, represented by the presence in the cytoplasm of erythrocytes, leukocytes, or phagocytic cell fragments, may be occasionally detected (Figure 12.60). The cells are either dispersed individually on the background or crowded around aggregates of hepatocytes, sometimes affected by nonspecific injury; in some cases extracytoplasmic cholestasis is detectable. Hemophagocytic sarcoma is characterized by more or less evident phenomena of erythrophagocytosis (Figure 12.61).

Generally, the recognition (or at least the suspicion) of a histiocytic neoplasm is fairly obvious on the basis of morphological appearance of the neoplastic cells. Although a complete description of histiocytic diseases is beyond the scope of this book, histiocytic sarcoma complex [57] encompasses a number of clinical entities, from interstitial dendritic cells origin, mostly represented by

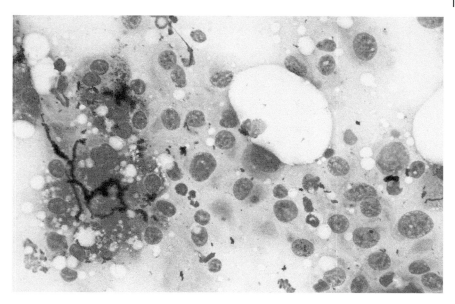

Figure 12.58 Liver, histiocytic sarcoma, FNCS, dog. Large, round to ovoid cells with slightly basophilic cytoplasm, sometimes containing clear globules; note the cholestasis in the sheet of hepatocytes on the left (MGG, 100×).

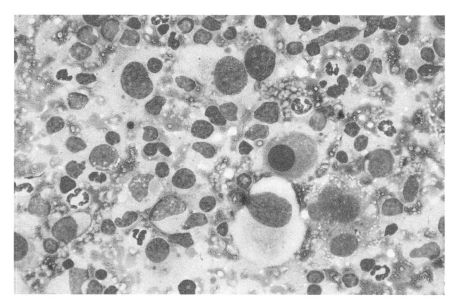

Figure 12.59 Liver, histiocytic sarcoma, FNCS, dog. Round to ovoid, sometimes indented nuclei show severe anisokaryosis and granular to clumped chromatin; cells on the right have multiple nuclei (MGG, 100×).

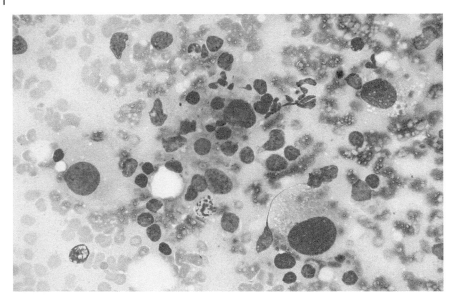

Figure 12.60 Liver, histiocytic sarcoma, FNCS, dog. Some neoplastic cells demonstrate cytophagocytosis (MGG, 100×).

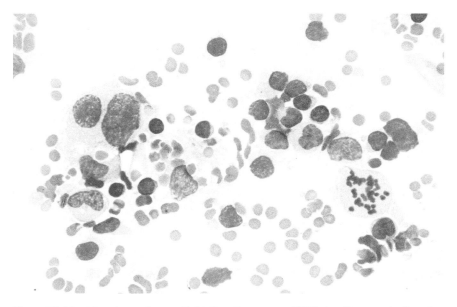

Figure 12.61 Liver, hemophagocytic histiocytic sarcoma, FNCS, dog. The neoplastic cells on the left show erythrophagocytosis; notice the atypical mitosis on the right (MGG, 100×).

histiocytic sarcoma, to bone marrow-derived macrophages, represented by hemophagocytic histiocytic sarcoma [58]. Histiocytic sarcoma may originate at a single site, called localized histiocytic sarcoma; when it spreads to distant sites, it is called disseminated histiocytic sarcoma. The liver is as likely to be involved as other organs, such as the spleen or lymph nodes, in disseminated forms of this neoplasm and, to the best of my knowledge, primary onset has not yet been described in the literature. Histiocytic sarcoma with liver involvement has also been described in cats [59].

12.3.8 Mast Cell Tumor

Cytomorphology: presence of intermediate to large round cells with cytoplasm filled with a variable amount of purple metachromatic granules (Figure 12.62). Depending on stain technique, the granules can be difficult to observe and are demonstrated by clumped, eosinophilic material; the nucleus is round with granular or compact chromatin; association of neoplastic cells with eosinophilic granulocytes is an infrequent finding; neoplastic mast cells tend to aggregate in more or less numerous groups, sometimes scattered on the background or thickened in groups in proximity to hepatocytes (Figure 12.63).

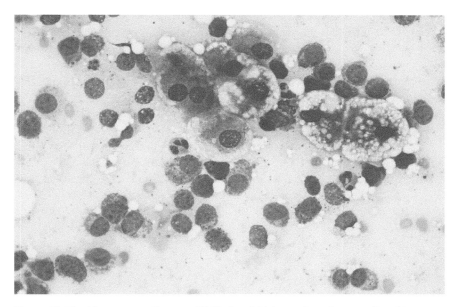

Figure 12.62 Liver, mast cell tumor, FNCS, dog. A high number of mast cells, with granulated cytoplasm, surround a small sheet of hepatocytes (MGG, 100×).

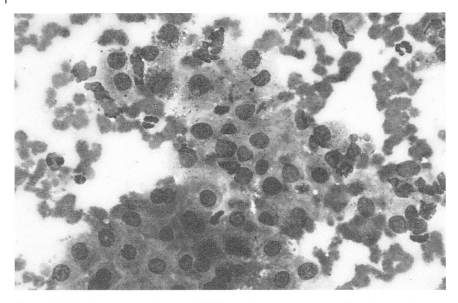

Figure 12.63 Liver, mast cell tumor, FNCS, dog. A large aggregate of poorly granulated, neoplastic mast cells crowded around a sheet of hepatocytes (MGG, 100×).

The hepatic localization of a large number of mast cells may be a marker of metastasis of primary cutaneous or mucocutaneous neoplasms, or part of visceral mastocytosis, a systemic mast cell disease which typically arises in the spleen. Dissemination of neoplastic mast cells in the liver is frequently preceded by primary cutaneous lesions and represents metastasis. Cytological evaluation of the liver should be included in staging of cutaneous mast cell tumors since ultrasonographic evaluation may be less useful in recognition of hepatic metastasis [60].

Clustering of neoplastic cells, compared with distribution as single scattered cells, should be considered a differential criterion for diagnosis of a liver localization of mastocytoma [61]. Unless they are present in large numbers, it is rather unlikely that single mast cells indicate involvement of the liver in a form of mastocytoma, and correlation with fibrosis and a form of chronic hepatitis must be investigated, since mast cells may be numerous when cytological features of fibrosis are detected (see Chapter 8). Moreover, neoplastic mast cells in liver demonstrate large size and a variable size and number of cytoplasmic granules, if compared with nonneoplastic mast cells which are small, with coarse granules.

Although rare, primary hepatic onset of mast cell tumor is possible and was previously described in a dog with a hepatosplenic lymphoma [62].

12.3.9   Hepatic Splenosis

This uncommon lesion, represented by multiple soft masses, arises when normal splenic tissue develops within the liver. This lesion may occur when splenic surgery or other traumatic causes introduce splenic tissue into the portal vein [63]. Although no cytological description of this disease has been reported, hepatic splenosis should be considered when polymorphic lymphoid population, together with hematopoietic cells, are observed in a smear from a hepatic nodule.

12.4   Metastatic Neoplasia

The liver is the most common organ to be involved in metastases, which are more common than primary neoplasms [7]. Consequently, when a primary malignant tumor has been recognized in abdominal organs, the presence of multiple liver nodules is probably due to a metastasis. Nevertheless, determining the origin of the primary tumor on the basis of morphological features can be difficult, and sometimes impossible, to do by cytological examination; a complete description of clinical and historical data, together with an accurate evaluation by imaging techniques, is necessary to correctly interpret the features of a neoplastic lesion of the liver.

Although the origin of hepatocellular proliferative diseases is easy to recognize, cholangiocarcinoma, mostly when widespread to the liver, can be confused with a metastasis from intestine, pancreas, kidney, prostate, mammary gland, or urinary bladder. A hepatic carcinoid may be confused with metastasis of a neuroendocrine tumor located elsewhere. Primary or metastatic sarcomas (mostly hemangiosarcoma, intestinal leiomyosarcoma or GIST) are much more difficult to recognize on the basis of morphological features and comparison with clinical and historical data is mandatory. Hepatic localization of a lymphoma and other round cell tumors must be differentiated by hepatic involvement of a generalized disease. From this point of view, many neoplastic lesions have to be compared with clinical and historical data in order to establish the presence of a primary hepatic tumor. In cases where a definitive diagnosis cannot be established, only a necropsy may help.

12.5 Criteria for Selection of Sampling Methods for Liver Nodular Lesions

If there are no preanalytical contraindications to the execution of the sampling procedure (coagulopathies or anesthetic risks), criteria for the choice of sampling methods between cytological and histological evaluation include the following.

- *Ease of collection*: cytological examination should always be the first choice in the evaluation of hepatic nodular lesions, especially when sampling by fine needle capillary suction (FNCS) is possible during ultrasound evaluation. The results provided by the cytological investigation can be used to produce a definitive diagnosis in several nodular diseases, including inflammatory suppurative septic lesions, hepatocellular carcinoma, both biliary and metastatic nonhepatocyte malign epithelial neoplasms (especially when the morphological features of the primary neoplasm are available), round cell neoplasms, and sarcomas.
- *Type of lesion*: nodular lesions of lacunar appearance mainly attributable to benign biliary neoformations (cholangioma) or vascular tumors (hemangioma, well-differentiated hemangiosarcoma) are difficult to evaluate cytologically due to the scarcity of material they release. Also, histological investigation has diagnostic relevance, but only if conducted on voluminous sections of tissue.
- *Diagnostic discrimination*: histopathological examination should be considered whenever the cell morphology is not sufficient to produce a definitive diagnosis and in the course of suspected malignant conditions. If cytological examination leads to suspecting a hyperplastic lesion, a hepatocellular adenoma, or a well-differentiated hepatocellular carcinoma, histopathological investigation could offer a conclusive diagnosis. However, it must be noted that the distinction between these lesions is based mainly on the characteristics of their marginal sections; in fact, a well-differentiated hepatocarcinoma can be identified and distinguished from a hyperplastic nodule or an adenoma on the basis of the architectural arrangements and infiltrative behavior toward the adjacent parenchyma. Therefore, sampling for histological investigation should be carried out on large sections, which can be obtained by complete resection of the lesion, as Tru-Cut® sampling may be inconclusive.
- *Identification of histotype*: a histopathological investigation may be necessary for the application of immunohistochemistry techniques on tissue sections when the distinction between similar neoplastic types (nonhepatocytic epithelial neoplasms of biliary or metastatic origin, sarcomas, round cell neoplasms) is necessary for clinical and therapeutic management, as well as for the formulation of a prognosis.

The diagnostic algorithm in Figure 12.64 provides procedural criteria based on the possible morphological aspects of a cytological sample acquired from solid hepatic nodular lesions. The indicated steps should be considered as general guidelines, to be subordinated to all possible morphological variables that may occur.

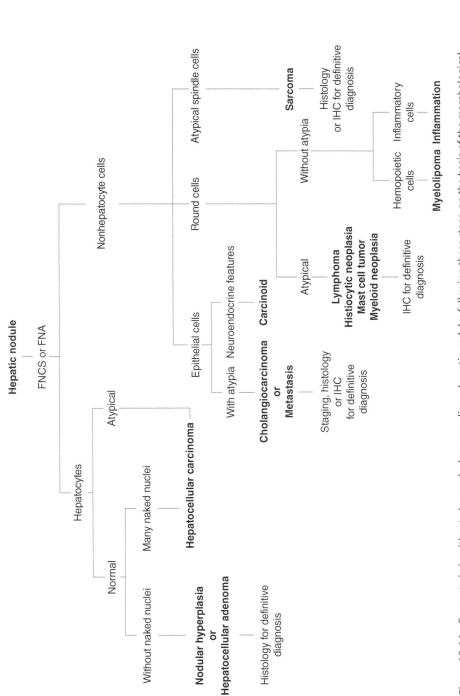

Figure 12.64 Suggested algorithm to be used when sampling a hepatic nodule; following these steps, on the basis of the morphological features of exfoliated cells, a neoplastic or nonneoplastic condition may be recognized.

12.6   Key Points

- Normal hepatocytes are indistinguishable from hepatocytes obtainedfrom nodular hyperplasia and hepatocellular adenoma. Comparison between cells from nodular lesions and from nonnodular liver may help in diagnosis.
- Most hepatocellular carcinomas are well differentiated; the classic cytological criteria of atypia are generally absent; the most reliable cytological feature is the presence of naked nuclei crowded around sheets of neoplastic hepatocytes.
- Neoplastic cells from cholangiocarcinoma may be indistinguishable from cells of malignant epithelial metastasis.
- Although large cell lymphoma or LGL lymphoma are easy to identify by cytology, small cell lymphoma in cats may share morphological features with lymphocytic inflammation.
- Neoplastic mast cells exfoliate frequently in small to medium-sized discohesive sheets. Single mast cells are much more likely to be normal or related to fibrosis.

References

1 Kemp, S.D., Panciera, D.L., Larson, M.M. et al. (2013). A comparison of hepatic sonographic features and histopathologic diagnosis in canine liver disease: 138 cases. *J. Vet. Intern. Med.* 27 (4): 806–813.

2 Warren-Smith, C.M.R., Andrew, S., Mantis, P., and Lamb, C.R. (2012). Lack of associations between ultrasonographic appearance of parenchymal lesions of the canine liver and histological diagnosis. *J. Small Anim. Pract.* 53 (3): 168–173.

3 Murakami, T., Feeney, D.A., and Bahr, K.L. (2012). Analysis of clinical and ultrasonographic data by use of logistic regression models for prediction of malignant versus benign causes of ultrasonographically detected focal liver lesions in dogs. *Am. J. Vet. Res.* 73 (6): 821–829.

4 Kanemoto, H., Ohno, K., Nakashima, K. et al. (2009). Characterization of canine focal liver lesions with contrast-enhanced ultrasound using a novel contrast agent-sonazoid. *Vet. Radiol. Ultrasound* 50 (2): 188–194.

5 O'Brien, R.T., Iani, M., Matheson, J. et al. (2004). Contrast harmonic ultrasound of spontaneous liver nodules in 32 dogs. *Vet. Radiol. Ultrasound* 45 (6): 547–553.

6 Bahr, K.L., Sharkey, L.C., Murakami, T., and Feeney, D.A. (2013). Accuracy of US-guided FNA of focal liver lesions in dogs: 140 cases (2005–2008). *J. Am. Anim. Hosp. Assoc.* 49 (3): 190–196.

7 Cullen, J.M. (2017). Tumors of the liver and gallbladder. In: *Tumors in Domestic Animals*, Ve, vol. 2017 (ed. D.J. Meuten), 604–605. Ames, IA: Wiley Blackwell.

8 Fabry, A., Benjamin, S.A., and Angleton, G.M. (1982). Nodular hyperplasia of the liver in the beagle dog. *Vet. Pathol.* 19 (2): 109–119.

9 Patnaik, A.K., Hurvitz, A.I., Lieberman, P.H., and Johnson, G.F. (1981). Canine hepatocellular carcinoma. *Vet. Pathol.* 18 (4): 427–438.

10 Trigo, F.J., Thompson, H., Breeze, R.G., and Nash, A.S. (1982). The pathology of liver tumours in the dog. *J. Comp. Pathol.* 92 (1): 21–39.

11 Masserdotti, C. and Drigo, M. (2012). Retrospective study of cytologic features of well-differentiated hepatocellular carcinoma in dogs. *Vet. Clin. Pathol.* 41 (3): 382–390.

12 Masserdotti, C., Rossetti, E., de Lorenzi, D. et al. (2014). Characterization of cytoplasmic hyaline bodies in a hepatocellular carcinoma of a dog. *Res. Vet. Sci.* 96 (1): 143–146.

13 Van Winkle, T., Cullen, J.M., van den Ingh, T.S.G.A.M. et al. (2006). Morphological classification of parenchymal disorders of the canine and feline liver – hepatic abcesses and granulomas, hepatic metabolic storage disorders and miscellaneous conditions. In: *Standard for Clinical and Histological Diagnosis of Canine and Feline Liver Disease* (ed. WSAVA Liver Standardization Group), 106–109. St Louis, MO: Saunders.

14 Nakanuma, Y. and Ohta, G. (1986). Expression of Mallory bodies in hepatocellular carcinoma in man and its significance. *Cancer* 57: 81–86.

15 Kelly, J.K., Davies, J.S., and Jones, A.W. (1979). Alpha-1-antitrypsin deficiency and hepatocellular carcinoma. *J. Clin. Pathol.* 32: 373–376.

16 Stromeyer, F.W., Ishak, K.G., Gerber, M.A., and Mathew, T. (1980). Ground-glass cells in hepatocellular carcinoma. *Am. J. Clin. Pathol.* 74: 254–258.

17 MacDonald, K. and Bedard, Y.C. (1990). Cytologic, ultrastructural and immunologic features of intracytoplasmic hyaline bodies in fine needle aspirates of hepatocellular carcinoma. *Acta Cytol.* 34: 197–200.

18 Nayar, R., Bourtsos, E., and de Frias, D.V.S. (2000). Hyaline globules in renal cell carcinoma and hepatocellular carcinoma. A clue or a diagnostic pitfall on fine-needle aspiration? *Am. J. Clin. Pathol.* 114 (4): 576–582.

19 Nyland, T.G., Koblik, P.D., and Tellyer, S.E. (1999). Ultrasonographic evaluation of biliary cystadenomas in cats. *Vet. Radiol. Ultrasound* 40 (3): 300–306.

20 Patnaik, A.K., Hurvitz, A.I., Lieberman, P.H., and Johnson, P.F. (1981). Canine bile duct carcinoma. *Vet. Pathol.* 18 (4): 439–444.

21 Maeda, A., Goto, S., Iwasaki, R. et al. (2022). Outcome of localized bile duct carcinoma in six dogs treated with liver lobectomy. *J. Am. Anim. Hosp. Assoc.* 58 (4): 189–193.

22 Roskams, T., de Vos, R., van den Oord, J.J., and Desmet, V. (1991). Cells with neuroendocrine features in regenerating human liver. *APMIS Suppl.* 23: 32–39.

23 Shiga, A., Shirota, K., Shida, T. et al. (1997). Hepatoblastoma in a dog. *J. Vet. Med. Sci.* 59 (12): 1167–1170.

24 Ano, N., Ozaki, K., Nomura, K., and Narama, I. (2011). Hepatoblastoma in a cat. *Vet. Pathol.* 48 (5): 1020–1023.

25 Loynachan, A.T., Bolin, D.C., Hong, C.B., and Poonacha, K.B. (2007). Three equine cases of mixed hepatoblastoma with teratoid features. *Vet. Pathol.* 44 (2): 211–214.

26 Manktelow, B.W. (1965). Hepatoblastoma in sheep. *J. Pathol. Bacteriol.* 89: 711–714.

27 Gold, J.R., Warren, A.L., French, T.W., and Stokol, T. (2008). What is your diagnosis? Biopsy impression smear of a hepatic mass in a yearling thoroughbred filly. *Vet. Clin. Pathol.* 37 (3): 339–343.

28 Prater, P.E., Patton, C.S., and Held, J.P. (1989). Pleural effusion resulting from malignant hepatoblastoma in a horse. *J. Am. Vet. Med. Assoc.* 194 (3): 383–385.

29 Dhaliwal, R.S., Johnson, T.O., and Kitchell, B.E. (2003). Primary extraskeletal hepatic osteosarcoma in a cat. *J. Am. Vet. Med. Assoc.* 222 (3): 340–342.

30 Jeraj, K., Yano, B., Osborne, C.A. et al. (1981). Primary hepatic osteosarcoma in a dog. *J. Am. Vet. Med. Assoc.* 179 (10): 1000–1003.

31 Chikata, S., Nakamura, S., Katayama, R. et al. (2006). Primary chondrosarcoma in the liver of a dog. *Vet. Pathol.* 43 (6): 1033–1036.

32 Kapatkin, A.S., Mullen, H.S., Matthiesen, D.T., and Patnaik, A.K. (1992). Leiomyosarcoma in dogs: 44 cases (1983–1988). *J. Am. Vet. Med. Assoc.* 201 (7): 1077–1079.

33 Park, J.W., Woo, G.H., Jee, H. et al. (2011). Malignant peripheral nerve sheath tumour in the liver of a dog. *J. Comp. Pathol.* 144 (2–3): 223–226.

34 Galofaro, V., Rapisarda, G., Lanteri, G., and Marino, F. (2008). Primary pleomorphic liposarcoma of the liver in a dog. *Pol. J. Vet. Sci.* 11 (4): 385–388.

35 Minkus, G. and Hillemanns, M. (1997). Botryoid-type embryonal rhabdomyosarcoma of liver in a young cat. *Vet. Pathol.* 34 (6): 618–621.

36 Hirao, K., Matsumura, K., Imagawa, A. et al. (1974). Primary neoplasms in dog liver induced by diethylnitrosamine. *Cancer Res.* 34 (8): 1870–1882.

37 Hayes, S., Yuzbasiyan-Gurkan, V., Gregory-Bryson, E., and Kiupel, M. (2013). Classification of canine nonangiogenic, nonlymphogenic, gastrointestinal sarcomas based on microscopic, immunohistochemical, and molecular characteristics. *Vet. Pathol.* 50 (5): 779–788.

38 Bertazzolo, W., Dell'Orco, M., Bonfanti, U. et al. (2005). Canine angiosarcoma: cytologic, histologic, and immunohistochemical correlations. *Vet. Clin. Pathol.* 34 (1): 28–34.

39 McCaw, D.L., da Silva Curiel, J.M., and Shaw, D.P. (1990). Hepatic myelolipomas in a cat. *J. Am. Vet. Med. Assoc.* 197 (2): 243–244.

40 Lombard, L.S., Fortna, H.M., Garner, F.M., and Brynjolfsson, G. (1968). Myelolipomas of the liver in captive wild Felidae. *Pathol. Vet.* 5 (2): 127–134.

41 Kamiie, J., Fueki, K., Amagai, H. et al. (2009). Multicentric myelolipoma in a dog. *J. Vet. Med. Sci.* 71 (3): 371–373.

42 Strombeck, D.R. (1978). Clinicopathologic features of primary and metastatic neoplastic diseases of the liver in dogs. *J. Am. Vet. Med. Assoc.* 173: 267–269.

43 Sumping, J.C., Maddox, T.W., Killick, D., and Mortier, J.R. (2022). Diagnostic accuracy of ultrasonography to detect hepatic and splenic lymphomatous infiltration in dogs and cats. *J. Small Anim. Pract.* 63 (2): 113–119.

44 Biller, D.S., Kantrowitz, B., and Miyabayashi, T. (1992). Ultrasonography of diffuse liver disease. A review. *J. Vet. Intern. Med.* 6 (2): 71–76.

45 Crabtree, A.C., Spangler, E., Beard, D., and Smith, A. (2010). Diagnostic accuracy of gray-scale ultrasonography for the detection of hepatic and splenic lymphoma in dogs. *Vet. Radiol. Ultrasound* 51 (6): 661–664.

46 Masserdotti, C. (2020). The cytologic features of biliary diseases: a retrospective study. *Vet. Clin. Pathol.* 49 (3): 440–450.

47 Warren, A., Center, S., McDonough, S. et al. (2011). Histopathologic features, immunophenotyping, clonality, and eubacterial fluorescence in situ hybridization in cats with lymphocytic cholangitis/cholangiohepatitis. *Vet. Pathol.* 48 (3): 627–641.

48 Roccabianca, P., Vernau, W., Caniatti, M., and Moore, P.F. (2006). Feline large granular lymphocyte (LGL) lymphoma with secondary leukemia: primary intestinal origin with predominance of a CD3/CD8(alpha)(alpha) phenotype. *Vet. Pathol.* 43 (1): 15–28.

49 Keller, S.M., Vernau, W., Hodges, J. et al. (2013). Hepatosplenic and hepatocytotropic T-cell lymphoma: two distinct types of T-cell lymphoma in dogs. *Vet. Pathol.* 50 (2): 281–290.

50 Suzuki, M., Kanae, Y., Kagawa, Y. et al. (2011). Emperipolesis-like invasion of neoplastic lymphocytes into hepatocytes in feline T-cell lymphoma. *J. Comp. Pathol.* 144 (4): 312–316.

51 Ossent, P., Stöckli, R.M., and Pospischil, A. (1989). Emperipolesis of lymphoid neoplastic cells in feline hepatocytes. *Vet. Pathol.* 26 (3): 279–280.

52 Rütgen, B.C., Flickinger, I., Wolfesberger, B. et al. (2016). Cutaneous T-cell lymphoma – Sézary syndrome in a boxer. *Vet. Clin. Pathol.* 45 (1): 172–178.

53 Valli, V.E., Bienzle, D., and Meuten, D.J. (2017). Tumors of the hemolymphatic system. In: *Tumors in Domestic Animals*, Ve (ed. D.J. Meuten), 279–280. Ames, IA: Wiley Blackwell.

54 Suwa, A. and Shimoda, T. (2018). Lymphoma-associated hemophagocytic syndrome in six dogs. *J. Vet. Med. Sci.* 80 (8): 1271–1276.

55 Stacy, N.I., Nabity, M.B., Hackendahl, N. et al. (2009). B-cell lymphoma with Mott cell differentiation in two young adult dogs. *Vet. Clin. Pathol.* 38 (1): 113–120.

56 De Zan, G., Zappulli, V., Cavicchioli, L. et al. (2009). Gastric B-cell lymphoma with Mott cell differentiation in a dog. *J. Vet. Diagn. Invest.* 21 (5): 715–719.

57 Moore, P.F. (2014). A review of histiocytic diseases of dogs and cats. *Vet. Pathol.* 51 (1): 167–184.

58 Moore, P.F., Affolter, V.K., and Vernau, W. (2006). Canine hemophagocytic histiocytic sarcoma: a proliferative disorder of CD11d+ macrophages. *Vet. Pathol.* 43 (5): 632–645.

59 Friedrichs, K.R. and Young, K.M. (2008). Histiocytic sarcoma of macrophage origin in a cat: case report with a literature review of feline histiocytic malignancies and comparison with canine hemophagocytic histiocytic sarcoma. *Vet. Clin. Pathol.* 37 (1): 121–128.

60 Pecceu, E., Serra Varela, J.C., Handel, I. et al. (2020). Ultrasound is a poor predictor of early or overt liver or spleen metastasis in dogs with high-risk mast cell tumours. *Vet. Comp. Oncol.* 18 (3): 389–401.

61 Stefanello, D., Valenti, P., Faverzani, S. et al. (2009). Ultrasound-guided cytology of spleen and liver: a prognostic tool in canine cutaneous mast cell tumor. *J. Vet. Intern. Med.* 23 (5): 1051–1057.

62 Akiyoshi, M., Hisasue, M., Asakawa, M.G. et al. (2022). Hepatosplenic lymphoma and visceral mast cell tumor in the liver of a dog with synchronous and multiple primary tumors. *Vet. Clin. Pathol.* 51: 414–421.

63 Knostman, K.A.B., Weisbrode, S.E., Marrie, P.A., and Worman, J.L. (2003). Intrahepatic splenosis in a dog. *Vet. Pathol.* 40 (6): 708–710.

Index

Please note that page references to Figures will be followed by the letter 'f', to Tables by the letter 't'